# Maternal and Child Health

*Edited by Miljana Z. Jovandaric*
*and Sandra Babic*

Published in London, United Kingdom

Maternal and Child Health
http://dx.doi.org/10.5772/intechopen.102240
Edited by Miljana Z. Jovandaric and Sandra Babic

Contributors
Olakunmi Ololade Ogunyemi, Hassan Taiwo Yahaya, Oluwakemi Mary Agoyi-Awoniyi, Zacharie Tsala Dimbuene, Tilahun Haregu, Paul-Denis Nzita Kikhela, Raphaël Muanza Nzuzi, Yoko Kato, Linda May, Filip Jevtovic, Arturo L. Delgado, Mfuneko Kopolo, Ernesto Rosales Gonzalez, Moeketsi Thabana, Luke Yamkela, Dumo Bangaza, Huseynova Saadat Arif, Panakhova Nushaba Farkhad, Orujova Pusta Ali, Hajiyeva Nurangiz Nizami, Hajiyeva Adila Sabir, Mukhtarova Sevinj Nabi, Agayeva Gulnaz Telman, Matthias Fischer, Anja Buschulte, Jamila Gurbanova, Afat Hasanova, Prema Subramaniam, Vitezslav Marek, Roman Zahorec, Stefan Durdik



First published in London, United Kingdom, 2023 by IntechOpen
IntechOpen is the global imprint of INTECHOPEN LIMITED, registered in England and Wales, registration number: 11086078, 5 Princes Gate Court, London, SW7 2QJ, United Kingdom

British Library Cataloguing-in-Publication Data
A catalogue record for this book is available from the British Library

Additional hard and PDF copies can be obtained from orders@intechopen.com

Maternal and Child Health
Edited by Miljana Z. Jovandaric and Sandra Babic
p. cm.
Print ISBN 978-1-80356-683-2
Online ISBN 978-1-80356-684-9
eBook (PDF) ISBN 978-1-80356-685-6

For EU product safety concerns:
IN TECH d.o.o., Prolaz Marije Krucifikse Kozulić 3, 51000 Rijeka, Croatia,
info@intechopen.com or visit our website at intechopen.com.

# Meet the editors

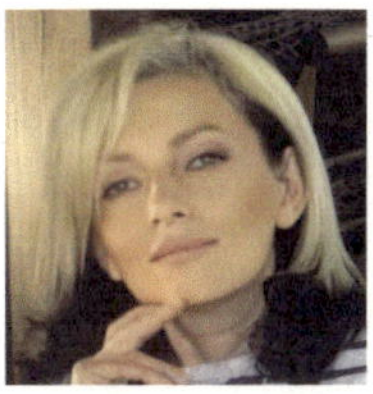

Miljana Z. Jovandaric graduated from the Faculty of Medicine, University of Belgrade, Serbia, in 1989, and completed a specialization in pediatrics at the University Children's Hospital, Belgrade, in 1999. She completed her specialization in Neonatology in 2003. Dr. Jovandaric completed her master's thesis in 2006 and her doctoral dissertation in 2018, both at the School of Medicine, University of Belgrade. She is the author and co-author of more than eighty-four scientific papers presented at national and international conferences and published in scientific journals. Dr. Jovandaric is currently head of the Department of Sick Newborns, Clinic for Gynecology and Obstetrics, Department of Neonatology, Clinical Centre of Serbia.

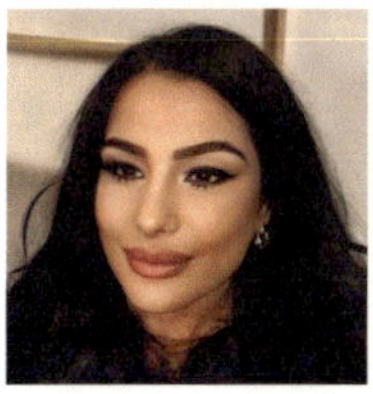

Dr. Sandra Babic graduated from the Medical Faculty, University of Belgrade, Serbia, where she also completed Specialist Academic Studies (SAS) in Human Reproduction. She is currently pursuing a doctorate in human reproduction, perinatology, and neonatology at the same university. She is a specialist in gynecology and obstetrics. Dr. Babic has published several works in national and international professional journals. She is also the author/co-author of thirty-two papers presented at domestic and foreign conferences. She currently works at the Department of Fertility Control, Clinic for Gynecology and Obstetrics, Clinical Centre of Serbia.

# Contents

# Preface

Maternal and child health is an important public health issue because we have the opportunity to end preventable deaths among all women, children, and adolescents and to greatly improve their health and well-being. Far too many women, infants, and children worldwide have little or no access to essential, quality health services and education, clean air and water, and adequate sanitation and nutrition. Factors influencing the development of diseases in women and children are many, depending on genetic factors, the way the child is born, the dietary habits of the mother during pregnancy, the use of antibiotics during pregnancy, and so on. Health depends on climate, lifestyle, diet, education, and ethnic and racial divisions, among other factors. Are we educated enough about health? How much do we know about how to be healthy? Is health a decision of our free will with less financial investment and more knowledge? Is health the art of living in harmony with nature or the disease of a modern society burdened with financial power?

**Dr. Miljana Z. Jovandaric and Sandra Babic**
Clinical Centre of Serbia,
Beograd, Serbia

Chapter 1

# Hydatid Cysts in Children

*Arturo L. Delgado, Mfuneko Kopolo, Dumo Bangaza, Ernesto Rosales Gonzalez, Luke Yamkela and Moeketsi Thabana*

## Abstract

Hydatid disease is one of the important health problems in developing countries. Can affect any part of the human body, it commonly affects lungs and liver. Because of poor data and preventive measures in Sub-Saharan Africa, cystic echinococcosis (CE) is regarded as endemic disease. This is a retrospective study of children ages of 3 to 12 years admitted in pediatric surgical unit at Nelson Mandela Academic Hospital (NMAH), from April 2015 to aril 2020. We studied groups of age, sex, organs affected, treatment and complications. We studied 56 children; the group of age most affected was 5 to 10 years, females accounted for 51.8%, and male for 48.2%, lung hydatid cysts in 44.6% of cases, 41.1% had liver cysts, 8.9% of the patients had cysts in multiple locations. In 46 cases (82%), the treatment was surgical: punction-aspiration-injection and respiration (PAIR) removing the germinal layer, following in the post operatory with Albendazole and Praziquantel. In 10 cases (18//%) was given only medical treatment. Females were most affected, and the lungs were the organs most affected followed by liver.

**Keywords:** hydatidosis, pair, CE, echinococus granulosus, echinococcosis

## 1. Introduction

The Echinococcosis is a zoonotic disease caused by a parasitic infection with the larval stage of the tapeworm Echinococcus genus [1]. Among the recognized species, two are of medical importance – E. granulosus and E. multilocularis – causing cystic echinococcosis (CE) and alveolar echinococcosis (AE) in humans respectively. Cystic echinococcosis is the most common form of the disease [2].

The Echinococcus can infect domestic animals, the adult tapeworms are carried by the definitive host (dogs) asymptomatically and can transmit the worms through defecation contaminating humans if ingest affected intermediate host meat (sheep, cattle, goats, and pigs). Human hydatid cyst is a health problem in some developing countries [3], this disease is usually asymptomatic for years until develop complications: such as compressive symptoms or rupture of the cyst causing anaphylactic shock. In most of the patients the symptoms are non-specific for the disease [4].

## 2. Course of infection

Have been reported in Ultrasound (US) surveys that the cysts may grow 1–50 mm per year or persist without changes according with [5, 6]; these cysts may spontaneously rupture or collapse and also disappear [5, 7].



IntechOpen

The sequence of the changes during the natural history of this cysts is not well define [8], the Liver cysts appear to grow at a lower rate than the lung cysts [6]. The symptoms appear in this disease usually when the cyst compresses or ruptures into neighboring structures [6].

The diagnosis of CE is based on symptoms when they are present, Ultrasound, CT imaging techniques, and serology. The Proof of the presence of protocolises could be given by microscopic examination of the fluid and histology [9].

Source: Expert consensus for the diagnostic and treatment of cystic and alveolar echinococcosis in humans, 2010 [5].

The ultrasound (US) examination is the basis for the diagnosis and the WHO classification of the disease in abdominal locations of the cysts, this technique could visualize cysts in other locations no suspected, such as lung when the cysts are located peripherally [9].

The WHO-IWGE classification; in 1995 standardized and allowed a natural grouping of the cysts into three relevant groups of CE [Cystic echinococcosis]: active, transitional, and inactive; this classification added a "cystic lesion" (CL), to Gharbi classification [9, 10].

The transitional cysts according with WORL HEALTH classification, can be differentiated into with detached endocyst and (predominantly solid with daughter vesicles. The inactive Cysts are late stages of the disease.

The Computed tomography (CT), magnetic resonance (MR) imaging, and cholangiopancreatography (MRCP) are indicated in [1] subdiaphragmatic location, [2] disseminated disease, [3] extra abdominal locations, [4] in complicated cysts (abscess, cysto-biliary fistulae) and [9] in some cases when is necessary in the pre-surgical evaluation. MRI imaging should be preferred to CT due to better visualization of liquid areas.

## 3. Serology of the echinococcus granuloses

According with some authors [9] the Sensitivity of the serum antibody detection using indirect hemagglutination, ELISA, or latex agglutination, in the hydatid cyst fluid antigens, is between 85 and 98% for liver cysts, 50–60% for lung cysts and 90–100% for multiple organ cysts.

Other cestode infections such as E. multilocularis and Taenia solium, malignancies, liver cirrhosis and presence of anti-P1 antibodies limits the Specificity of all those tests due to this possibility, so a confirmatory test should be used as: (arc-5 test; Antigen B (AgB) 8/12 kDa subunits or EgAgB8/1 immunoblotting) [9].

Any organ could be affected by Echinococcal cysts, including the muscles but the commonest organs affected are lungs, liver, and spleen. If the liver is affected, might cause a compartmental abdominal Syndrome, and might cause obstructive jaundice when there is compression to the biliary system. When the lungs are affected, the patients could present with productive cough, weight loss and poor appetite (**Figures 1** and **2**).

Rupture of the cyst into pleural cavity can with shortness of breath and on chest x-ray it can be confused with pleural effusion, that could wrongly make the doctors to insert a chest drain into the cyst for mistake, founding later in another chest x-ray/or CT-chest a cystic cavity [5, 6, 8] (**Figure 3**).

The main aim of our study was to find out the prevalence of the Hydatid Cysts in children and found up the organs more common affected in children.

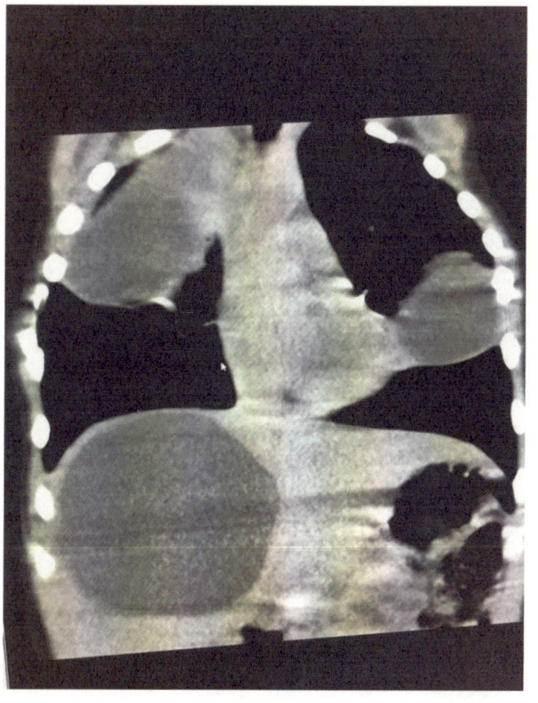

**Figure 1.**
*Hydatid cysts in the liver and left lung. Source: Author's record.*

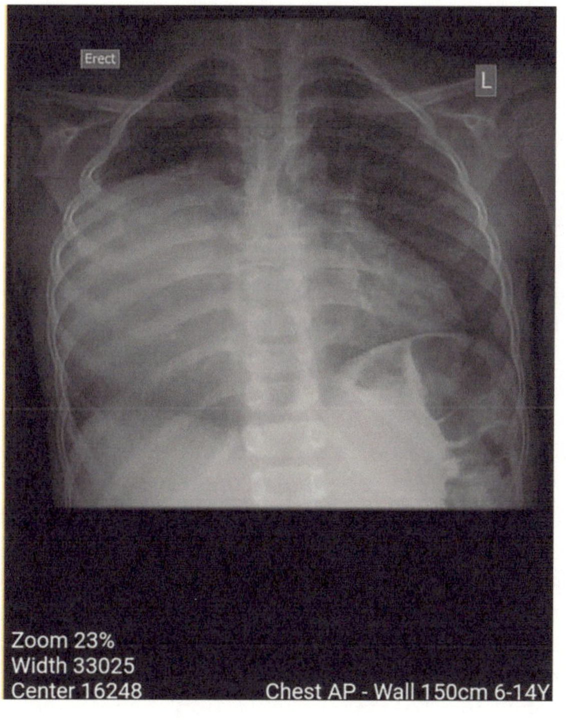


**Figure 2.**
*Hydatid cyst right lung lower lobe. Source: Author's record.*

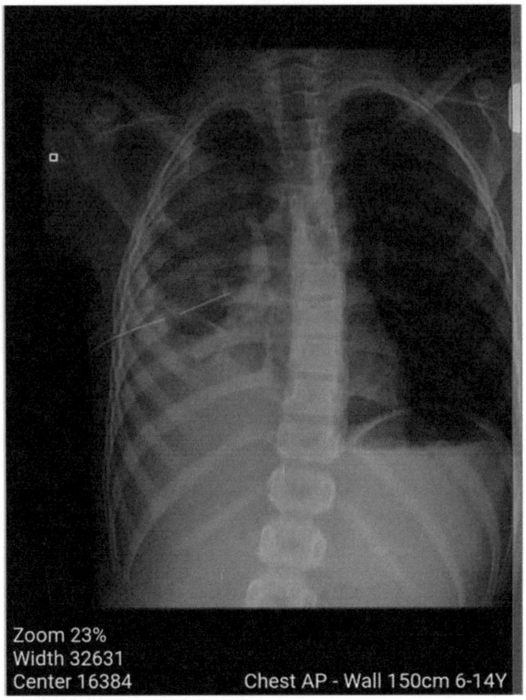


**Figure 3.**
*Intercostal drainage into a cyst cavity of a hydatid cyst in the right lung, mistakenly for parapneumonic pleural effusion. Source. Author's record.*

## 4. Method

We performed a retrospective study of every child of 3 to 12 years of age admitted in our surgical pediatric ward (N 56), suffering from hydatid cyst. We studied patients with this diagnosis from April 2015 to April 2021. Were studied 56 patients: analyzing the age, sex, localization of the cyst, treatment, and complications. The diagnosis was based on clinical history, physical examination, serology test, abdominal ultrasound, chest X ray, Computer Tomography (CT) and histology. The ultrasound ad CT scans were the most useful investigations in the diagnostics.

The decision to perform a surgical treatment was based on the size of the cyst when it was 6 cm or more, and when the patient having compressive symptoms and signs of complicated hydatid cyst. In hydatid cysts on the liver the compressive symptoms and sings were jaundice, itchiness, abnormal liver function testes; In Hydatid cyst on the lung; the patient could present productive cough, shortness of breath, when there is a bronchial communication, and ruptured of the cyst to the pleural cavity.

Patients with hydatid liver cyst and those with lung hydatid cysts where was showed in the CT no communication of the cyst cavity to a bronchus were performed PAIR (puncture – aspiration- injection and re aspiration, through laparotomy and thoracotomy on those with cysts in the lung. Was use 5% hypertonic saline solution for the injection considering that this concentration of the saline solution is enough to kill the Ovo's; after the PAIR, the cyst was opened and removed the germinal layer (endocyst) and taken it for histopathology examination as a confirmation of the disease; a capitonage was done in every cyst and a drain was let in the cystic cavity. In case of lung hydatic cyst was let an intercostal drain into the cyst cavity and also into the pleural space.

In the post-operative time, we continued the children with Albendazole (20-50 mg/kg/day) and Praziquantel (30-40 mg/kg/day) for 3 months; depending on the resolution of the cysts in some cases the Albendazol was given more than 3 months, depending on the result of the liver function tests performed monthly to rule out hepatic toxicity.

Patients with hydatid cyst size of 5 cm or less, and with no signs of compression or any other complications were treated conservatively with the combination of Albendazole and Praziquantel this treatment was given for 3 months or more depending on the resolution of the cysts.

Full Blood Count and liver function test were performed before the initiation of the treatment and every month after starting with medical treatment to find out drug toxicity.

## 5. Results

Were analyzed 56 children, 25 of them (44.6%) had Cysts in the liver, 23 (41%) had lung Cysts. Some patients 8.9% had cysts affecting liver, lung, spleen and in other organs shown in **Table 1**.

As it can be seen in the **Table 1**, the most affected group of age was the one of patients from 5 to 10 years for 52% of the patients, the group of children with more than 10 years was the second in frequency with 36%.

The presentation of hydatid cysts in liver were more frequent in male with 28.6% than in females 16%; on the other hand; lung hydatid cysts were more frequent in female affecting 26.8%, as is showing in **Table 2**.

In 40 cases (70%) was performed a surgical treatment (PAIR and enucleation of the endocyst); in 27% of the patients with Lung Hydatid cysts to whom were performed this procedure developed in the post operatory a bronchus pleural fistula that closed by Itself mostly in the first week (**Table 3**).

In 18% of our cases the treatment was medical treatment without surgery during a period of 6 to 8 months, expressed in **Table 4**.

| | **Liver Hydatic** | | **Lung Hydatic** | | **Soft Tissue** | | **Multiple** | | **Total** | |
|---|---|---|---|---|---|---|---|---|---|---|
| **Ages** | **No** | **%** | **No** | **%** | **No** | **%** | **No** | **%** | **No** | **%** |
| < 1 year | — | — | — | — | — | — | — | — | — | — |
| 1–5 years | 5 | 8.9 | 2 | 3.6 | 0 | 0 | 0 | 0 | 7 | 12.5 |
| 5–10 years | 12 | 21.4 | 17 | 30.4 | 0 | 0 | 0 | 0 | 29 | 51.8 |
| > 10 years | 8 | 14.3 | 4 | 7.1 | 1 | 1.8 | 7 | 12.5 | 20 | 35.7 |
| Total | 25 | 44.6 | 23 | 41.1 | 1 | 1.8 | 7 | 12.5 | 56 | 100 |

*Source: Patient files.*

**Table 1.**
*Patients' age vs. organs location of the cyst.*

| Gender | Cyst Location | | | | | | | | | |
|---|---|---|---|---|---|---|---|---|---|---|
| | Liver Hydatic | | Lung Hydatic | | Soft Tissue | | Multiple | | Total | |
| | No | % | No | % | No | % | No | % | No | % |
| Male | 16 | 28.6 | 8 | 14.3 | 1 | 1.8 | 2 | 3.6 | 27 | 48.2 |
| Female | 9 | 16.1 | 15 | 26.8 | 0 | 0.0 | 5 | 8.9 | 29 | 51.8 |
| Total | 25 | 44.6 | 23 | 41.1 | 1 | 1.8 | 7 | 12.5 | 56 | 100.0 |

*Source: Patient files.*

**Table 2.**
*Cysts location vs. gender.*

| Complications | Liver Hydatic | Lung Hydatic | Soft Tissue | Total | |
|---|---|---|---|---|---|
| | No | No | No | No | % |
| Biliary Fistula | 1 | | | 1 | 1.8 |
| Bronchopleural Fistula | | 15 | | 15 | 26.8 |
| Wound infection | | | 1 | 1 | 1.8 |
| Total | 1 | 15 | 1 | 17 | 30.4 |

*Source: Patients files.*

**Table 3.**
*Complications vs. cyst's location.*

| Treatment | | | | | | |
|---|---|---|---|---|---|---|
| | PAIR | | Medical alone | | | Total |
| | N | % | N | % | | 100% |
| Patients | 46 | 82 | 10 | 18 | 56 | |

*The histopathology examination of the germinal layer confirmed the echinococcus granulosus.*

**Table 4.**
*Patient vs. treatment performed.*

## 6. Discussion

In endemic countries the Hydatid disease is still a national health problem and needs prevention for its eradication or its control [3]. Symptoms of hydatid disease depend on which organs are affected and only are evident when the complications arise, but most patients with hydatid cysts are asymptomatic, and the diagnosis is usually made incidentally during clinical or radiological examination for unrelated reasons [11, 12].

In our study of 56 cases, 29 (52%) were females and 27 (48%) were males in other studies the statistical analyses indicate that in children males are more likely to be infected with lung hydatid, while females were infected more with liver hydatid cysts [9, 13], result found also in our study; in total we found that the hydatid cyst disease in our children was no significative differences of affectation between the liver 41% and the lung 45%.

Hydatid cyst can affect any organ, but the two organs most involved are liver and lungs. The involvement of lungs, liver and other organs in the same patient in our study accounted in 8.9% of the cases.

The group of age commonest affected was from 5 to 10 years, in 32 patients (64%).

In human hydatid cysts Echinococcus granulosus is the most common cause as it was in our children, confirmed with histopathology of the endocyst (germinal, layer) this finding were also reported by other authors [13–17].

## 7. Conclusions

The incidence of hydatid disease in children increase with age.

The organs more frequently involved were liver and lungs.

As can be affected for hydatid cyst in the same patient lung and liver, we recommend that when a hydatid cyst of the liver is diagnosed a chest x-ray should be done to rule out lung involvement specially in endemic regions.

The most common cause of human hydatid cyst is the Echinococcus granulosus as it was diagnosed with echinococcus Elisa and confirmed with endocyst (germinal layer) taken for histopathology.

In most case a conservative surgical technique (PAIR) and total or partial enucleation of the endocyst is sufficient, followed by medical treatment post operatively with Albendazol and Praziquantel for no less than 3 months.

## Author details

Arturo L. Delgado[1*], Mfuneko Kopolo[1], Dumo Bangaza[1], Ernesto Rosales Gonzalez[2], Luke Yamkela[1] and Moeketsi Thabana[1]

1 Department of Surgery, Walter Sisulu University (WSU)/Nelson Mandela Academic Hospital (NMAH), Umtata, Eastern Cape, South Africa

2 Department of Family Medicine and Rural Health, Walter Sisulu University (WSU)/ Nelson Mandela Academic Hospital (NMAH), Umtata, Eastern Cape, South Africa

*Address all correspondence to: delgadoarturo15@yahoo.com

## References

[1] Larriu E. Prevention and Control of Hydatidosis at Local Level South American Initiative for the Control and Surveillance of Cystic Echinococcosis. 2017. Available from: https://iris.paho.org/handle/10665.2/49043

[2] Albadawi AAM. Role of serology and histopathology in diagnostic of human cystic echinococcosis. Journal of AIDS and HIV Infections. Available from: http://www.annexpublishers.co/full-text/JAHI/4203/Role-of-Serology-and-Histopathology-in-Diagnostic-of-Human-Cystic-Echinococcosis.php/. Received: June 29, 2018; Accepted: December 18, 2018; Published: December 21, 2018

[3] Mirshemirani A, Khaleghnejad A, Kouranloo J, Sadeghian N, Rouzrokh M, Hasas-Yeganeh S. Pediatric Surgery Research Center, Mofid Children's Hospital, Shahid Beheshti University of Medical Sciences, Tehran, Iran. Received: Jul 11, 2010; Final Revision: Jan 12, 2011; Accepted: Mar 02, 2011

[4] Botezatu C, Mastalier B, Patrascu T. Hepatic hydatid cyst – diagnose and treatment algorithm. Journal of Medicine and Life. 2018;**11**(3):203-208

[5] Romig T, Zeyhle E, Mchperson CN, Rees PH, Were JB. Cyst growth and spontaneous cure in hydatid disease. Lancet. 1986;**1**:861

[6] Frider B, Larrie E, Odriozola M. Long term outcome of asymptomatic liver hydatidosis. Journal of Hepatology. 1999;**30**:228-231

[7] Wang Y et al. Post-survey follow-up for human cystic echinococcosis in northwest China. Acta Tropica. 2006;**98**(1):43-51. DOI: 10.1016/j.actatropica.2006.01.009. PMID: 16676417

[8] Rogan TM et al. Hydatid cysts: Does every picture tell a story? Trends in Parasitology. 2006;**22**(9):431-438. DOI: 10.1016/j.pt.2006.07.003

[9] Brunetti E, Kern P, Vuitton DA. Expert consensus for the diagnosis and treatment of cystic and alveolar echinococcosis in humans. Acta Tropica. 2010;**114**(1):1-16. DOI: 10.1016/j.actatropica.2009.11.001. ISSN 0001-706X

[10] Gharbi HA et al. Ultrasound examination of the hydatic liver. Radiology. 1981;**139**:459-463

[11] Ramos G, Orduña A, Garcaí-Yuste M. Hydatid cyst of the lung: Diagnosis and treatment. World Journal of Surgery. 2001;**25**(1):46-57

[12] Santivanez S, Garcia HH. Pulmonary cystic echinococcosis. Current Opinion in Pulmonary Medicine. 2010;**16**(3):257-261. DOI: 10.1097/MCP.0b013e3283386282

[13] Velasco-Tirado V et al. Recurrence of cystic echinococcosis in an endemic area: A retrospective study. BMC Infectious Diseases. 2017;**17**:455. DOI: 10.1186/s12879-017-2556-9

[14] Zhang W, Wang S, McManus DP. Echinococcus granulosus genomics: A new dawn for improved diagnosis, treatment, and control of echinococcosis. Parasite. 2014;**21**:66

[15] Sumer A, Caglayan K, Altinli E, Koksal N. Case report: Spontaneous liver hydatid cyst rupture in a child, Israel. The Journal of Emergency Medicine. 2009;**9**(I):13, 14-16

[16] Talaiezadeh A, Maraghi S. Hydatid disease in children: A different pattern than adults. Pakistan Journal of Medical Sciences. 2006;**22**(3):329-332

[17] Bulent K, Gultekin G, Serdar H, et al. Analysis of pulmonary hydatidosis according to their segmentary location. Clinical Pulmonary Medicine. 2008;**15**(1):8-12

Chapter 2

# Hygiene Aspects of Premature Nutrition

*Matthias Fischer and Anja Buschulte*

## Abstract

The very low birth weight and the not fully developed immune system make preterm infants especially susceptible to infections. Therefore microbiological food safety of preterm nutrition is a particular challenge. This is also due to the fact that breastfeeding is often not possible in these infants. There are several obstacles to breastfeeding, such as intensive care conditions and individual nutritional requirements of the newborn. The chapter covers the microbiological aspects of preterm nutrition, including quality requirements for commercial infant formulas, breastmilk fortifiers and extracted breast milk. The main pathogens of concern (e.g. *Cronobacter* spp. *Salmonella* spp. and *Clostridium botulinum*) are discussed in detail, including related food safety indicators. An important part of the chapter is devoted to the hygienic aspects of preterm formula preparation techniques, storage conditions and microbiological risks linked to certain feeding techniques (e.g. tube feeding). The risks associated with microorganisms found in commercial infant formula and in the prepared environment, as well as the risk of biofilm formation, are described. Options and requirements for risk mitigation are discussed in detail.

**Keywords:** hygiene, food safety, *Cronobacter* spp., premature nutrition, microbiological contaminants

## 1. Introduction

The very low birth weight and the not fully developed immune system make preterm infants especially susceptible to infections. The development stage of the organ systems depends stringently on the gestation age of the newborn. This concerns also the intestinal tract and the immune system. Both are especially important for the resilience of infants to gastrointestinal infections. Regarding the intestinal tract, different aspects have a crucial influence on the immune defence. One critical aspect is that in mammals antibodies cannot pass the placenta. The newborn receives the first antibodies with the first milk of the mother, which is especially immunoglobulin enriched. Under circumstances of a mature digestion, proteins of the size of an immunoglobulin (150 to 1 Mio kDa) cannot pass the intestinal wall to enter the bloodstream. Therefore, the gut of mammals shows a different anatomy during their first days of life than the gut of adult individuals. The tight junctions seal usually the gaps between the enterocytes. These seals are quite open for the first three to four days of life to enable the antibodies of the colostrum to pass into the bloodstream.

Although this is not necessary for human neonates, the mechanism is still observed phylogenetically and is even more pronounced in preterm infants. These open tight junctions provide an option for microorganisms and toxins like endotoxins to enter the bloodstream unhindered [1, 2].

Unlike the offspring of other mammals, immune globulins of primate species can pass the placenta and are present in the bloodstream of infants immediately after birth. This has the advantage that the colostrum in humans is not an absolute requirement for the survival of the newborn. However, the antibody-enriched colostrum also provides human infants with humoral protection against intestinal infections during the first days of life. In premature births, the breastmilk is often not available or does not meet the nutritional requirements of the preterm infant and definitely does not provide the quality of a fully developed colostrum [1, 2].

The virulence of microorganisms depends on the ability to overcome the non-specific and specific immune barriers of the host organisms, followed by the effect of specific pathogen factors, like toxins, on the target organ system or tissue. As explained before the specific and non-specific immune defences in very young infants are underdeveloped and weak. The lack of humoral immune protection is compounded by the underdeveloped acid barrier in the stomach of young children. This means pathogenic microorganisms can reach the small intestine, from where they can enter the blood system without passing the usual barriers. Thus, even bacteria with low virulence can cause significant harm to these premature organisms [1, 3].

The intestinal flora is competitive against pathogens that have reached the intestine, which provides an additional protection against gastrointestinal infections. Young children still need to develop their body flora including the gut flora. Their gut flora is not stable in the perinatal period [1]. Until now, it was assumed that the body of the newborn is sterile and that only during birth the first bacteria will colonise the skin and the enteral tract. For some years now, it has been discussed whether the fetus already comes into contact with microorganisms intrauterine [1, 4]. In any case, birth itself plays a decisive role in the colonisation of the body of the infant, as bacteria from the mother are transmitted intensively to the baby during the birth procedure [1]. Preterm infants are often not born in the natural way but by caesarean section. This way of birth already shows a retarded and different type of intestinal colonisation in term infants and is even more critical in preterm infants with regard to the formation of the intestinal microbiome.

The low birth weight and the awkward ratio of body surface to body weight make neonates more susceptible to toxin effects and low infection doses of microorganisms [5]. Moreover, the metabolic functionality in preterm infants is often not fully developed, which influences the neutralisation, turn over and excretion of bacterial toxins [6].

These special conditions meet the specific nutritional requirements of the preterm infants, often requiring individual formulas. In many cases, breastfeeding is not possible or has to be provided with extracted milk fortified with certain ingredients, and even the application of feeding tubes is also a regularly applied praxis. This requires specific hygiene precautions in the preparation, storage and application of food for preterm babies.

## 2. Types of preterm feedings

There are different types of formula designed for preterm infants. However, the most preferable option is the feeding of breastmilk. Due to the shortened gestation period, the breastmilk of the mothers alone is often not sufficient for the nutritional needs of the preterm child and certain supplements (breast milk fortifiers, thickeners) have to be added [1]. The addition of powdered breastmilk fortifiers to the liquid milk bears significant hygiene risks. The breastmilk fortifiers are not sterile but have similar microbiological properties as powdered formula. The feeding practices of breastmilk to preterm infants is another hygiene issue. Direct breastfeeding is usually not possible for these patients, so milk is applied by tube feeding, syringes or baby bottles. The extraction and storage of the breastmilk pose several hygiene risks, with the addition of fortifier being only one of many other contamination sources.

In many cases, breastmilk is not available or specific nutritional needs require the use of infant formula products. From a hygiene point of view, the use of sterilised ready-to-feed formula is the most recommendable option. If used as a sole source of nutrition, the contamination risks during handling and feeding are minimised. The sterilisation process guarantees the inactivation of all infectious microorganisms including spore-forming bacteria and viruses. However, the bacterial debris of these inactivated microorganisms is still in the formula but the amount is very low due to the advanced hygiene standard during the manufacturing process. A quality parameter for this kind of formula is the level of endotoxin. Endotoxins are lipopolysaccharides, which can be found as part of the cell wall of gram-negative bacteria. The group of gram-negatives includes *Enterobacteriaceae*, but also the non-fermenters, which are often detected as water bacteria in process water. Endotoxins in food are usually not an issue, as the transfer from the gut into the bloodstream is very limited. The tight junctions between the enterocytes seal the enteron very effectively, and the small amount of endotoxins, which still pass the intestinal wall, are efficiently neutralised in the liver. In young infants and especially in preterm infants, the situation is different. On one hand, the tight junctions are still open as explained earlier and on the other hand, the detoxification ability of the liver is not fully developed. If the level of endotoxins in the formula is too high, these lipopolysaccharides can enter the bloodstream. Monocytes would recognise them and start a cytokine-mediated immune response. These endotoxin levels can cause symptoms from mild sub-clinical disorders to febrile temperature. As the health status of preterm infants is quite fragile in many cases, the endotoxin-related burden is an additional factor that could influence the development of the newborn.

Powdered formula for preterm infants is available in a range of formats to meet the broad variety of the nutritional needs of prematurely born babies. Basically, the conventional starter formulas are also applicable for preterm infants. However, based on their gestational development stage, the responsible medical staff has to decide about the requirement of individually tailored diets. A variety of vitamin, mineral protein and calorie enriched formulas and fortifiers are available on the market to meet the individual nutritional needs of preterm infants. In some cases, the under-developed gastrointestinal tract of the baby is not able to break down proteins and carbohydrates, so the infant has to be supplied with free amino acids. In many cases, reflux might be a problem, which requires the addition of thickeners to the diet. These products are often combined or added to breastmilk or ready-to-feed formula.

Powdered infant formula is manufactured under the highest hygiene standards but is not sterile. The microbiological burden of the powder is usually low, but the reconstituted formula is an optimal growth medium where bacteria can multiply rapidly. The powdered formula differs from conventional milk powder in its composition. From a microbiological point of view, the elevated fat content is most important, because it protects bacteria in the dry environment and promotes the biofilm formation on contact surfaces. The powdered formula is produced in several steps based on milk ingredients like skim milk powder and whey protein concentrate. These ingredients have been spray dried and are usually delivered as bulk products to the baby food manufacturer. The spray drying process is conducted in a counter flow of falling droplets against a hot air stream of more than 70°C. However, the bacteria in the droplets are protected against high temperatures due to the evaporative cooling. Therefore, spray drying is not a sufficient heat treatment to kill off microorganisms. These bulk ingredients are mixed with a range of specific nutrients like minerals, vitamins and lipids. The dosing of the especially important micro-ingredients is often done manually and bears a certain risk of contamination from the operating staff. Fat blends are often stored at higher temperatures, which make the survival of vegetative bacteria impossible, but the introduction of bacteria spores can be linked to this type of ingredient. The blending and packing operation of the baby powder is usually a fully automated step, nevertheless, contamination risks are not fully excluded. There are a number of bacteria species, which have adapted to the dry environment and are found as process contaminants in many powder factories.

The intestinal flora is an important part of the defence against gastrointestinal infections and plays an irreplaceable role in digestion and metabolism. The gut flora is labile in all infants during the first 12 months of life, but in preterm infants, this is an issue of special concern. The underdeveloped intestinal flora is seen as a factor that increases the risk for necrotising enterocolitis (NEC) and late-onset sepsis (LOS) [7]. The addition of probiotic strains to the diet of preterm infants is widely discussed. In a number of randomised clinical trials, the prophylactic effect against NEC has been shown and no adverse effects of the probiotics have been reported [8]. It is not clear whether the risk for NEC is only significantly reduced in preterm infants who receive breastmilk supplemented with probiotics. An advantage is not observed in infants fed with probiotic-enriched formula. It seems that there is a shortage of some bioactive ingredients in the formula, which are present in breast-milk [7]. However, the risk of probiotic sepsis remains one of the concerns linked to this kind of supplementation, especially in preterm infants [9–12]. Invasive diseases linked to probiotics are reported rarely and have never been seen in a randomised clinical trial [8]. However, 49 case reports on invasive diseases in children caused by probiotics have been published in the scientific literature between 1995 and 2021 according to D'Agostin et al. [9]. About 55% of the cases occurred in preterm infants and the majority developed septicaemia. All kinds of probiotics were involved in cases of invasive disease. In most cases, the outcome was favourable but in three cases there was a fatal outcome caused by *Limosilactobacillus reuteri* (formerly *Lactobacillus reuteri*), *Saccharomyces boulardii* and *Bacillus clausii* [9].

Therefore, the use of probiotics in preterm infants requires a careful assessment of benefits and risks for the individual case. Important risk factors for probiotic bacteremia are e.g. intestinal comorbidity and intravenous catheters [9].

Full-term infants who are exclusively breastfed usually have no need for additional liquid supply [13]. The fluid and electrolyte management of preterm infants is much more complex and in most cases, glucose solutions and water are supplied. In Europe, however, it is common practice to feed newborn infants herbal teas to supply the baby with fluid and relieve intestinal colic, although herbal teas are not recommended for young infants because they impair iron absorption due to the polyphenols they contain [13].

Furthermore, herbal teas often contain high levels of different bacteria species that are not eliminated during preparation and teas serve as an excellent growth medium for microorganisms.

## 3. Microbiological contaminants in preterm feed

Microorganisms get into the preterm feed from different sources. Some originate from dairy ingredients and survived the different processing steps. These bacteria are, in most cases, spore formers and can survive high temperatures, but *Enterococci* may also survive the processing steps along the entire line. Another important contamination route are blending operations in powdered infant formula manufacture. A specific flora of microorganisms has become adapted to the dry environment in powder production facilities. These bacteria can survive in the powdered formula for a long time. A high risk of contamination is posed by bacteria that get into the formula during preparation. The germs have the opportunity to multiply rapidly in the dissolved formula. These microorganisms may come from the hands of the person preparing the formula, from insufficiently cleaned feeding equipment or from the environment.

In 2004, microbiology experts categorised potential pathogens, based on the available evidence of a clear link between infant illness and the presence of certain pathogens or bacterial toxins in powdered infant formula. Three categories have been defined, from category A (clear evidence of causality) over category B (causality plausible, but not yet demonstrated) and C (causality less plausible, or not yet demonstrated). Only *Salmonella* spp. and *Cronobacter* spp. were identified as bacteria with a clearly proven link between illness and formula contamination [14].

*Salmonella* spp. are gram-negative rods. Their natural reservoir is the intestinal tract of animals. *Salmonella* shows a temperature range for growth from 5–45°C with an optimum temperature between 35° and 42°C [15, 16]. A pH below 4.0 reduces the number of viable *Salmonella* cells. Therefore, the acid barrier of the stomach forms an effective line of defence against *Salmonella* infections. Infants have a higher pH in the stomach than adults and the milk-based diet further protects against *Salmonella* during the gastric passage. This makes infants and premature babies especially vulnerable to *Salmonella* infections [17, 18]. A heat treatment of 2 minutes at 70°C sufficiently kills *Salmonella*. They are not able to form spores [19].

*Salmonella* causes severe gastrointestinal infections with diarrhoea, abdominal pains, chills, fever, vomiting and dehydration. The onset of symptoms is usually within 72 h. The severity of the disease depends, among other things, on the virulence of the *Salmonella* strain and the amount ingested, but all serotypes are potentially pathogenic to humans. Infants and especially preterm infants are among the most vulnerable individuals, where even small infectious doses of less than 100 cfu can lead to potentially fatal infections [16, 19, 20].

*Cronobacter* spp. formerly known as *Enterobacter sakazakii* belongs to the genus *Enterobacteriaceae* [21]. The growth optimum of the microorganism is between 25° and 45°C. There is no multiplication below 5° C and over 45° C [22]. Under optimal growth conditions, the generation time is about 20 minutes and drops to 2 h at room temperature [23].

In dry environments, *Cronobacter* spp. can survive up to 2 years [24, 25]. The reservoir of *Cronobacter* spp. includes a wide variety of environmental and food sources [26–29]. Biofilm formation was observed on different surfaces, which is particularly important for the hygiene management in the care environment of preterm infants [23, 30]. *Cronobacter* spp. infections are rare and occur especially in neonates and very young children. Since 1958, reports on about 180 infections have been published [31]. In 95% of all *Cronobacter* cases, infants are affected during their first 2 months of life and the risk for infections is particularly high for preterm infants [31]. *Cronobacter* spp. cause meningitis, septicaemia and NEC [32–34].

Between 20 and 80% of the infants do not survive a *Cronobacter* infection [32–34]. Among those who recover from the disease, many suffer from lifelong sequelae [31]. The infection dose, for Cronobacter infections, is estimated to be between 100 and 10,000 bacterial cells per meal [35]. This makes bacterial growth in the prepared food a necessary prerequisite for an infection, because these high numbers of Cronobacter cells are not reached in any kind of formula or extracted breastmilk. Although powdered infant formula is in most cases the source of the infection, it has to be regarded that the bacterium can also derive from utensils for formula preparation like bottles or teats, water and handling failures [31]. Biofilm formation is a risk factor for *Cronobacter* infections if feeding is done via stomach tubes for medical purposes [30, 31, 36]. Stojanovic et al. (2011) analysed 150 herbal teas and found 32% of the teas *Cronobacter*-positive [37]. Teas are part of the usual diet even of very young infants as early as the first week of life [38]. The teas are often kept over hours at the bedside of babies or patients and are used for oral hygiene or perfusion of stomach tubes [39, 40]. This makes teas a potential *Cronobacter*-infection risk.

Microorganisms for which World Health Organisation (WHO) experts see a causality between powdered infant formula and infections, but which has not yet been proven, are summarised in category B [14]. These are:

*Pantoea agglomerans, Escherichia vulneris, Hafnia alvei, Klebsiella pneumoniae, Citrobacter koseri, Citrobacter freundii, Klebsiella oxytoca, Enterobacter cloacae, Escherichia coli, Serratia spp., and Acinetobacter spp.*

Besides these species, other members of the *Enterobacteriaceae* have been reported to cause gastrointestinal infections such as *Edwardsiella trada, Proteus mirabilis, Providencia alcalifaciens, Morganella morganii, Moellerella wisconsensis* [16].

The group comprises *Enterobacteriaceae* with a known potential for opportunistic infections, which makes them particularly important for vulnerable patients like young children and preterm infants. The category has been extended to *Acinetobacter* spp., which does not belong to the genus *Enterobacteriaceae* but is regarded as a similar hazard for nosocomial infections. Category B has similarity to the so-called bile tolerant gram-negative bacteria (BTGNB), a method- and risk-based classification that is used by the US Pharmacopoeia. The BTGNB group includes all gram-negative bacteria that grow in the presence of bile salts and can utilise glucose [41]. The most important species in this group is *Escherichia (E.) coli*, which includes a number of enteropathogenic variants.

The other listed species include more particular pathotypes [36].

All *Enterobacteriaceae* are thermolabile and a rather mild heat treatment at 70°C over 2 min will eliminate them if the initial levels do not exceed an amount, which is usually assured by general hygiene measures. However low levels of *Enterobacteriaceae* can be expected in powdered infant formula even when these products have been manufactured according to all hygiene requirements. These nosocomial pathogens require fairly high infection doses (e.g. $10^8$ and $10^{10}$ cfu per g for enterotoxic *E. coli* in adults) to cause illness [42]. In many cases, the infections are linked to tube feeding or catheter treatment. In most cases, multiplication of these bacteria in the feed is necessary to reach the necessary dose for oral infections. This group of bacteria is often involved in the formation of biofilms [43, 44] which are a particular risk in constant feeding via tubes where giving sets can harbour biofilms. A feed contaminated with high numbers of bacteria poses a significant risk for handling contamination of intravenous catheters, which might cause a septicemic infection.

*E. coli* is a member of the family of *Enterobacteriaceae*. The term coliforms, which is often found in this context, comprises a larger group of *Enterobacteriaceae* that have the ability to form acid from lactose and glucose. The group of coliforms includes *E. coli*, *Citrobacter* spp., *Klebsiella* spp., *Enterobacter* spp. and others [19, 45].

*E. coli* is part of the intestinal flora of humans and animals. *E. coli* indicates, therefore, faecal contaminations [45]. Usually, *E. coli* strains found in the human bowel are harmless commensals but an increasing number of sero- and pathotypes have been identified to be linked to diarrhea and, in some cases, severe complications [45]. A broad range of symptoms has been described, next to diarrhoea, fever, headache, abdominal spasm and nausea. Several types of pathogenic *E. coli* exist with different pathomechanisms based on adhesins, toxins, invasion proteins and defence mechanisms against host immunity. The main *E. coli* pathogen groups are:

Enteropathogenic *E. coli* (EPEC), which are an important causative agent of diarrhoea in infants and young children under 1 year of age with fever, vomiting or abdominal pain. Incubation times of 17 to 72 hours have been reported. The illness lasts between 6 hours and 72 hours. The adhesions structures bundle forming pili (Bfp) and the intimate attachment (EaeA-gene coded) are the underlying patho-mechanisms. EPEC generally do not produce any enterotoxins. A destruction of the intestine brush border microvilli (attachment and effacing lesions) is the consequence of the infection.

The Enteroaggregative *E. coli* (EAEC) carry a plasmid that enables them to produce fimbriae, short pilus-like structures that promote specific aggregation and adherence of the bacteria to the gut cells.. The EAEC are able to produce a heat-stable enterotoxin. These features result in a prolonged diarrhoea of more than 14 days, especially in children [19].

Enteroinvasive *E. coli* (EIEC): The illness caused by this group develops within 2–48 hours. The EIEC strains invade the cells of the large intestine. Typical symptoms are bloody and non-bloody diarrhoea or dysentery with fever, headache, muscular pain and abdominal spasm [19].

Enterotoxic *E. coli* (ETEC): ETEC colonises the small intestine but do not enter the host cells. They produce toxins of a heat-labile and a heat stable type. The strains cause diarrhoea in infants but can also be pathogenic for adults, presenting as travellers diarrhoea. The infection dose in adults is about 108 to 1010 cells and for infants some log units lower [19, 42].

The Enterohemorrhagic *E. coli* (EHEC) are also known as Verotoxin or Shiga-like-toxin producing *E. coli* (VTEC or STEC, respectively). The strains attach to the cells of the large intestine and cause lesions and bloody hemorrhagic colitis, the produced toxins (verotoxin, enterohemolysin) enter the bloodstream to cause kidney failure (hemolytic uremic syndrome - HUS) and can damage the blood cells (thrombotic thrombocytopaenic purpura - TTP). The detection of the Shiga toxin gene indicates always the potential of an EHEC infection including HUS and TTP. These diseases are very severe and particularly in infants, the risk of a fatal outcome or permanent kidney failure is high. The infection doses have been reported as low as 10 cells. The incubation period may range from 3 to 9 days and duration of the illness from 2 to 9 days. EHEC are able to survive pH 2, which enables them to pass the gastric acid barrier [16, 19, 45].

A number of other pathogenic *E. coli* cause diseases of the urogenital system, meningitis and sepsis. These strains are usually not spread through the consumption of food [16, 46].

In category C, WHO experts included microorganisms for which they considered the causal relationship to be less plausible or for which it has yet not been possible to demonstrate that there is a stringent link between infant infections and powdered formula. In some cases, infections in infants were reported but the concerned microorganism has not been isolated from infant formula, in other cases, the bacterium has been found in infant formula but was not linked to illness in infants. However, these organisms are well-known food pathogens and there is no reason that infants would not share the risk of other vulnerable groups [14]. The category C organisms are:

> *Bacillus cereus, Clostridium perfringens, Clostridium difficile, Clostridium botulinum, Listeria monocytogenes, Staphylococcus aureus, and coagulase-negative Staphylococci.*

*Bacillus (B.) cereus* is a spore-forming bacterium and a well-known enteropathogen. It appears as gram-positive rod and is able to grow aerobically and anaerobically [47]. Some strains produce different toxins: a heat-sensitive enterotoxin, which causes diarrhea and is formed in the small intestine, although preformation in food is also possible. The extremely heat stable emetic toxin (cereulide) is performed in the affected food and causes an intoxication with symptoms occurring within 1 to 5 hours. The symptoms last for up to 24 h with nausea, vomiting and occasional diarrhoea. The numbers of bacteria cells found in food associated with *B. cereus* poisoning have usually been as high as $10^6$ $g^{-1}$. However, occasionally numbers as low as $10^3$ $g^{-1}$ were observed and should be regarded as a potential risk for infants especially. In most cases of *B. cereus* intoxication, a storage of the food at elevated temperatures made an excessive growth of the bacterium in the food possible and resulted in a preformation of toxins. The heat stability of the emetic toxin bears the risk that during bacterial growth emetic toxin is formed and subsequent process steps reduce the *B. cereus* counts, but the toxin concentration remains at high levels. A classical microbiological analysis would not reveal the problem. The toxins are detectable only with more elaborated methods [45]. *B. cereus* is found in a wide range of environmental and food sources like soil, dust, surface water, cereals, milk and dairy products. *B. cereus* has been found in 9–12% of fresh milk and in 35–87% of pasteurised milk samples. In powdered milk, *B. cereus* is a common contaminant and 50% of the powdered infant formula was found to be positive for *B. cereus* on low levels (10–100 $g^{-1}$). While this does not pose an acute risk, problems can occur if there is temperature abuse or prolonged storage time after reconstitution of the formula, which allows bacteria to grow to higher numbers [16, 48]. Bacteria of the B. *cereus* group have a growth range between 10 and 50°C, with an optimum temperature of 28–35°C. Some psychotropic strains are capable to grow at 4°C. The minimum pH of growth is 5.5, below 4.5 vegetative cells start to die off [16]. *B. cereus* spores are heat resistant and can, therefore, be expected after spray-drying of milk-based infant formula.

In newborn and preterm infants, clinical manifestations such as septicemia, respiratory tract infection, enterocolitis, hepatitis, endocarditis, endophthalmitis and encephalitis with cerebral abscess have been reported in infections with *B. cereus*. The severity of these infections in neonates ranges from symptomless gut colonisation to fatal outcomes in 40% of the cases. The role of bacterial exotoxins in these diseases is not clear [49]. Infection with *B. cereus* in infants is rare but severe. Between 1977 and 2018 only 50 cases have been reported in the scientific literature. In most cases, the source of infection has not been proven and there have been suspicions about respiratory support equipment, umbilical catheterization, gastric feeding tubes, dried formulas, extracted human breastmilk, linens, heating, ventilation and air conditioning systems [50]. Although the link between infection and extracted human breastmilk has never been proven, *B. cereus* remains a major concern in the hygiene management of both extracted breast milk and infant formula. About 10% of the breastmilk bank amount is discarded in 9 of 10 cases due to contamination with *B. cereus*. Standard procedures for extracted human breastmilk handling include a pasteurisation step at 62.5°C for 30 min but *B. cereus* in spore form can survive this treatment. Additionally, a post-pasteurisation contamination is possible as *B. cereus* is often found in the hospital environment [49].

*Clostridia* are gram-positive rods that grow only under strictly anaerobic conditions [19]. They are found ubiquitously in air, soil, water, faeces, milk and other foods [16, 45]. Foodborne illnesses can be caused by several species, including *Clostridium (Cl.) perfringens, Cl. botulinum Cl. butyricum, Cl. sphenoides, Cl. sordelli, Cl. spiroforme, Cl. difficile and Cl. baratii* [45].

*Cl. perfringens* has been found in low numbers in many types of processed food and is part of the physiological gut flora in low numbers. *Cl. perfringens* is able to grow at unusually high temperatures. The optimal growth temperature is 43–45°C where the generation time is rather short (7 minutes). The growth temperature range reaches from 15 to 50°C. The pH optimum for growth is quite narrow and stretches from pH 6 to 7; very little growth occurs below pH 5 or above pH 8.3 and in the presence of oxygen [16]. *Cl. perfringens* enterotoxins can cause food poisoning. Viable vegetative cells in large numbers (>$10^5$ $g^{-1}$) in foods are necessary for foods to cause food poisoning [16]. The toxin is normally formed in the human intestine. Onset of symptoms is 8–24 hours after ingestion of the contaminated food. The illness causes diarrhoea and severe abdominal pain. A full recovery is normally seen within 24 h. Complications and death from *Cl. perfringens* have been reported among vulnerable consumers. In preterm infants, the bacterium has been linked to NEC. About one-third of the preterm neonates have been seen colonised 3 weeks after birth. A colonisation was unlikelier with prolonged breastfeed, antibiotic treatments and oxygen support. The positive effect of breastmilk has been seen only for breast-fed infants and infants fed with extracted milk from their own mother. In pasteurised donor milk, the effects have not been observed [16, 51]. An antibiotic treatment can also cause imbalances of the gut flora causing severe health problems caused by *Cl. perfringens* or *Cl. difficile. Cl. difficile* belong to the normal gut flora but may cause also severe symptoms in neonates like diarrhoea with dehydration and electrolyte imbalance, abdominal pain and distension and poor weight gain sometimes with fatal outcome.

*Cl. botulinum* is much less often found then *Cl. perfringens. Cl. botulinum* is able to form seven different toxins. Responsible for most human botulism cases are the toxins A, B, E and F to lesser extent. There is a mesophilic group that is proteolytic and able to produce heat-resistant spores and a psychotropic group, which is often non-proteolytic and whose spores have only a low heat resistance [16]. Growth is seen from 20 to 40°C under strictly anaerobic conditions. The toxins of *Cl. botulinum*, which are pre-formed in food, initially cause vomiting and diarrhoea after ingestion and end with double vision, difficulty in breathing and paralysis. The toxins work by interference with nerve stimuli. The *Cl. botulinum* toxin is the most potential natural poison. Its lethal dose varies between 0.005 and 0.5 μg. 0.1 g of food in which *Cl. botulinum* has grown is sufficient to cause botulism [16, 45, 52].

A special form of botulism is infant botulism which may be caused by the ingestion of only a few spores. These multiply in the gut of the infant and produce toxins. The disease causes progressive paralysis that starts with constipation and develops into respiratory paralysis and death if untreated. The illness affects only infants below 1 year of age. Adults are protected by their normal, inhibitory gut flora. Infant botulism has been caused by honey in which 80 spores $g^{-1}$ were present [53].

In 2001, the case of a 5-month-old infant with infant botulism with a possible link to powdered infant formula has been reported. *Cl. botulinum* type A was found in faeces. In a powdered infant formula package fed to the baby and an unopened package of the same batch *Cl. botulinum* type B has been found. Therefore, no stringent link could be made between the formula and the illness but the case shows that infant feed is a potential source for infant botulism [54, 55].

*L. monocytogenes* is a non-sporing, gram-positive rod. The bacterium is facultatively anaerobic with growth temperatures from 1 to 45°C and a growth pH between 4.6 and 9.2. The range for optimal growth is 30 to 37°C and a pH of 7. It can cause listeriosis with symptoms such as fever, headache, gastrointestinal problems and vomiting, which can develop into meningitis or septicaemia, especially in vulnerable groups like neonates. Pregnant women may develop a flu-like disease, which could cause miscarriage or diaplacentar can harm the foetus. The infection can reach mortality rates of 30 to 40% in vulnerable groups. An infection dose of $10^6$–$10^9$ cells is necessary to cause infections in immunocompromised persons. However, in most cases, the human infections with L. monocytogenes remain clinically inapparent. Foods involved in the foodborne infections are raw milk products, raw vegetables and meat products. Pasteurisation temperatures can kill *Listeria* reliably, therefore a contamination of powdered infant formula from raw materials is unlikely but a recontamination from the environment remains possible [45]. In neonates, a listeriosis is seen in two forms. The granulomatosis infantiseptica listeriosis is an intra-uterine acquired infection with early onset (< 7 days of life). The incubation time for a listeriosis infection ranges between 3 and 70 days [45]. The onset of symptoms (fever, respiratory, circulatory and liver distress) of the early onset infection is usually seen within 2 days after birth. A second form is the late onset listeriosis with symptoms like hyperexcitability, vomiting, cramps and pneumonia. This infection is acquired during birth from the mother or after birth from the environment. *Listeria* infections can be transmitted directly in person-to-person contact or via food or other vehicles. Nevertheless, to our knowledge, a transmission with infant feed has not been reported so far [56, 57].

*Staphylococcus (S.) aureus* is a gram-positive coccus, which can grow aerobically or anaerobically. *S. aureus* grows between 7 and 48°C, with an optimum of 35–37°C and a pH range from 4.0 to 9.8 (optimum 6.0–7.5). *S. aureus* is inactivated by pasteurisation [45]. The bacterium can cause food intoxication when a heat stable enterotoxin is produced. The toxin is performed in the food when the bacteria have the chance to grow to high numbers. *Staphylococci* are poor competitors and do not grow well in the presence of other microorganisms. In food with considerable numbers of competitive flora, the presence of *S. aureus* may be unproblematic [16]. However, infant feed is a food with a very low bacterial flora, which gives contaminants, such as *Staphylococci,* enough room to multiply. There are eight different enterotoxins types, which can be produced by *S. aureus*. Most common in food intoxication is enterotoxin A. 0.1 to 1 µg toxin in food can cause food poisoning [16, 19, 45]. The enterotoxin production is linked to the bacterial growth and the amount of toxin produced depends on the strain and growth conditions (pH, temperature, water activity). Levels of $10^5$–$10^6$ cells per g of food have to be reached for relevant toxin concentrations. The symptoms of *Staphylococcus*-intoxication include nausea, vomiting, abdominal spasm and diarrhoea and headache and muscle spasm. The symptoms start abruptly within 2–8 hours and recovery is normally seen within a few hours [16, 45].

In food microbiology, the focus is on coagulase positive *Staphylococci* which also include *S. intermedius* and *S. hyicus*. These two species can produce the enterotoxins also. The methicillin-resistant *Staphylococci* (MRSA) are a topic of concern in the health care environment. MRSA have the same potential to produce enterotoxins as any methicillin-sensitive strain. In 2002, an outbreak of gastrointestinal illness has been linked to MRAS for the first time [58].

In very low-birthweight neonates infections with coagulase negative *Staphylococci* are a matter of concern. These *Staphylococci* are responsible for more neonatal infections than *S. aureus. S. epidermidis* is the predominant species in these infections but there are also reports of neonatal infections with *S. haemolyticus, S. hominis, S. warneri, S. saprophyticus, S. cohnii* and *S. capitis* [14, 59, 60].

The reservoir of *S. aureus* and other *Staphylococci* is the human mucosa in the nose and throat. *S. aureus* can be found on the nasopharyngeal mucosa of 20–40% of the healthy population in Germany and the Netherlands. The bacteria are often transferred by handling food from the skin of the operators [18, 45].

## 4. Microbiological quality parameters of infant food

Powdered infant formula is manufactured under high-standard hygiene conditions. Therefore, the products have an extremely low bioburden but are not sterile. To control the microbiological quality of the powders, quality parameters have been laid down in different legislations and recommendations. The European legal standards consist of three types of parameters. These are, on the one hand, direct tests for pathogens or safety criteria (*Cronobacter, Salmonella, Listeria, S. aureus, B. cereus, E. coli and C. perfringens*) and, on the other hand, the following two process hygiene criteria:

a. the index microorganisms that point to the possible occurrence of pathogenic organisms in foods (*Enterobacteriaceae,* sulphite reducing *Clostridi*a).

b. indicator organisms that are used for the validation and control of the process integrity and hygiene (total viable count (TVC), yeast and moulds and *Enterococci*).

The pathogens have been discussed in detail above. Quality control tests for *Salmonella* and *Cronobacter* are required in most legislations. Commission Regulation (EC) No 2073/2005 [46] requires to prove the absence of *Salmonella* in 30 times 25 g and *Cronobacter* in 10 times 30 g for dried infant formula and products for special medical purposes for infants under 6 months of age. Additionally, ready-to-eat foods for infants are required to be negative for *L. monocytogenes* in 10 times 25 g.

Similar requirements are found in a number of national and international standards. For *Cronobacter* and *Salmonella* criteria identical to the Commission Regulation (EC) No 2073/2005 [46] are found in the Codex Alimentarius documents [61] and the US-FDA requirements [62].

The process hygiene criteria are used to indicate the possible presence of an underlying contamination with severe pathogens. The Commission Regulation (EC) No 2073/2005 [46] has defined process hygiene criteria. Presumptive *B. cereus* is an indicator for toxigenic *B. cereus,* which has to be tested 5 times in 1 g (counts exceeding 500 cfu/g are not acceptable but one sample with counts between 50 and 500 cfu/g is accepted). *Enterobacteriaceae* have to be absent 10 times in 10 g. The presence of *Enterobacteriaceae* indicates an elevated risk for the presence of nosocomial pathogens of the BTGNB-group including *Salmonella* and *Cronobacter*. The Commission Regulation (EC) No 2073/2005 [46] lays it in the hands of the infant formula manufacturer to prove a stringent link between *Enterobacteriaceae* and *Cronobacter*. If this is possible, parallel tests for both species are not required as long as tests for *Enterobacteriaceae* are negative.

Another group of bacteria with index function are sulphite reducing *Clostridia* (SRC). The bacteria are gram-positive anaerobic rods and can reduce sulphite to H2S, which is of interest as an analytical characteristic for differentiating *Clostridia* from competing flora. The SRC are used as indicators for pathogenic *Clostridia*. These microorganisms are spore formers and can survive heat treatments such as pasteurisation steps. Therefore, the SRC also serve as good indicators of the microbiological quality of the processed raw materials [63]. The International Commission on Microbiological Specifications for Foods (ICMSF) regards SRC as a valuable parameter to indicate pathogenic *Clostridia*. A proposed limit of 100 cfu/g could show that the established hygiene control measures are sufficient to keep the risk for *Cl. botulinum* negligible [64].

*Enterococci* are used as an indicator bacterium for faecal contamination, often together with *E. coli* or coliforms. In powdered infant formula, *Enterococci* can be a useful indicator for severe hygiene failures as they have a higher heat resistance than gram-negative non-spore-forming rods and may reflect better the hygiene history of the production and raw material quality. Moreover, *Enterococci* are opportunistic pathogens and might pose a direct health hazard to vulnerable consumer groups like preterm infants [65]. *Enterococci* are usual contaminants in powdered infant formula and do not pose a direct health hazard in low numbers [66]. Elevated levels of *Enterococci* might indicate shortages in the production or handling hygiene of infant feed.

An obvious link between process and handling hygiene provides the total aerobic plate count. If elevated total aerobic plate counts are found this may be due to the poor quality of raw materials, inadequate cleaning of processes, the growth of microorganisms during manufacturing or recontamination after heat treatment. The Codex Alimentarius committee recommends a microbiological limit for mesophilic plate count of 5000 cfu/g with five samples to be tested of which two are allowed to range between 500 cfu/g and 5000 cfu/g [61].

The count of yeast and mould can support the assessment of the process quality. These microorganisms are found in powdered formula in small numbers, and numbers exceeding 100 cfu/g might indicate a hygiene problem [67]. A number of moulds are able to produce toxins, which could be e.g. carcinogenic. Therefore, an elevated level of moulds in the powdered formula is always a matter of concern.

## 5. Hygiene aspects in handling infant food

Certain microorganisms can survive the manufacturing process of powdered infant formula and may be present in low concentrations. Although the bacteria are not able to proliferate in the formula, some of them may remain viable for a long time. In addition, pathogens can also get into the formula afterwards, e.g. through contaminated preparation utensils or through inadequate hygiene. In turn, bacteria can multiply quickly in the ready-prepared formula if it is not properly cooled. Therefore, infant starter formula should be fed directly after preparation (i.e. within 2 hours) [68]. This recommendation applies in private households without exception.

Boiled drinking water has to be used for infant formula for children during their first months of life. Local sources of water contamination as well as long holding times of the water in pipes or the formation of biofilms on taps can result in higher levels of microbes and pathogens even in drinking water. Sterile filters are sometimes used as an alternative to the boiling of water. However, a recontamination may take place downstream of the filter. The process of boiling water serves to reduce and eliminate microbial risks but at the same time can lead to additional health risks to the infant, such as scalding or burn injuries. Feeding insufficiently cooled formula can cause scalding in the mouth of the infant. In order to avoid the latter, a few drops of the prepared formula from the baby bottle should be applied to the inside of the wrist to test the temperature. These drops of formula should not feel warm and certainly not hot. If the temperature control is done with thermometers, the contamination risk has to be regarded. Therefore, the use of a contactless infrared thermometer is recommended. The widespread practice of parents testing the temperature by drinking the infant's formula by themselves has to be avoided since a transfer of microbes from the oral flora of the parents to the infant will occur and that could later cause problems such as dental caries. The general hygiene criteria for the preparation of powdered infant starter formula also apply to preterm infants who have reached the stage where they can be fed in the same way as full-term infants. The handling requirements must also be complied with after the discharge from the hospital in private households, childcare facilities and daycare centres.

In the professional care environment (e.g. in day nurseries or hospitals) some deviating practices have been established like the preparation of larger quantities of formula in advance if preparation just before consumption is not possible. However, this approach requires an effective hygiene regimen and precise temperature monitoring. Sterile (aseptic) conditions are required in the facility used for preparation, and both the storage and transportation of the prepared formula must be temperature-controlled (no more than 24 hours at below 5°C) [68]. For these reasons, the preparation of formula in advance should only be practised in a professional environment, and even here, the alternative option of using commercial sterile liquid formula should be considered, since the storage of prepared infant formula always involves a greater risk [68].

When mixing powdered infant formula with water, the temperatures specified by the manufacturer must be strictly observed. Water temperatures ranging from roughly 20–50°C are appropriate for preparation. The formula must have cooled down to drinking temperature before feeding. The following hygiene rules must be observed during preparation [69]:

- Washing the hands thoroughly with soap and hot water (under a running tap) before preparation

- Thoroughly cleaning of bottles, spoons and teats with detergent and hot water, and afterwards proper drying. Boiling these utensils or immersing them in boiling water for at least 2 minutes provides an extra level of safety. The use of a commercial steriliser for baby bottles is also an option. These kinds of heat deactivation techniques are especially recommended for the care of infants, which have been born prematurely and in professional childcare environments.

- Powdered infant formula must never be prepared at the same time or space with the preparation of other foods, especially raw foods. A separation from equipment cleaning activities has to be applied as well.

- Powdered milk formula has to be stored in a dry, cool place and sealed tightly. Additional information is provided by the manufacturer.

- The bottles should only be prepared shortly before feeding and cooled to drinking temperature as quickly as possible (max. 15 min) to avoid the proliferation of microbes.

- The feeding should be finished within 2 hours and any remains of prepared formula have to be disposed of immediately.

- If a formula is allowed to dry in the equipment, cleaning is much more difficult. Therefore, bottles and teats should be rinsed with drinking water directly after use.

- Measuring scoops should be stored separately from the powder in a closed container and touched only by the handle. If the scoop is provided in the powder, it should be removed from the package with a clean set of tweezers.

- As an alternative to a formula preparation in advance for occasions like feeding infants at night, travelling with infants or preparing daily portions of formula for later feeding in childcare facilities, the best approach is to portion the powder into clean and dry bottles, store the boiled drinking water in a clean and sealed thermos flask and mix both only shortly before feeding. Professional childcare facilities like hospitals have particular strict conditions for the preparation of formula, they make a storage at below 5°C for a maximum of 24 h possible. The formula has to be portioned into separate bottles under the same strict hygiene condition immediately after preparation. Before storing in the refrigerator, the bottles have to be cooled down to room temperature as quickly as possible e.g. under running water. In such cases, the refrigerator temperature must be documented at regular intervals. At temperatures above 5°C, slow but constant bacterial growth is possible in the formula.

- Additives like fortifiers have to be added immediately before feeding if necessary.

- When brought to drinking temperature (max. 37°C) with a bottle warmer as fast as possible (max. 15 min) the formula can be fed to the infant within 2 hours. These temperatures offer ideal conditions for bacterial growth during prolonged feeding.

Preterm infants require special care and a high hygiene standard during their first days or weeks of life. The infants are usually nursed in hospitals during this critical period. In the hospital environment, special hygienic requirements have to be met. Therefore, it is recommended to establish a dedicated milk preparation room [70]. The hygiene requirements for the milk preparation room should be described in detail in a hygiene plan that covers the following aspects as a minimum [69]:

Structural requirements:

- The milk preparation room should be a defined environment with conditioned air (defined temperature and humidity). Only authorised staff should get access to the milk preparation room, so access has to be regulated. The staff has to be trained on hygiene rules on a regular basis. The traffic routes in the facility have to be defined to minimise the risk of cross-contamination. A one-directional flow from powdered formula to the prepared bottles or feeding containers is recommended and crossing traffic of waste, formula for disposal or equipment for cleaning with prepared formula and sterilised equipment has to be avoided. The handling of fresh formula should be organised in a "white" area which is separated from the grey area used for the handling of bottles and equipment for cleaning.

Equipment:

- The equipment for use has to be defined. For extremely critical techniques like tube feeding, one-way material should be used consequently. This kind of material is for single use only and must not be reused. This applies also to relatively short time frames. The materials have to be disposed of in a way that a mix-up with new unused material and unintended reuse can be excluded. Re-useable material has to be cleaned in a validated cleaning procedure.

Procedures:

- A risk assessment for the different types of feed should be done. There are types of feed with elevated hygiene risks like tube feeding and unfreezing and supplementing extracted human milk. The procedures for preparation must be specified in detail. A picture board is recommended to illustrate the different preparation procedures for the staff. The preparation of especially critical feeds can be done under a laminar airflow. Tools for risk management like a HACCP (Hazard Analysis Critical Control Point) concept should be applied and a detailed documentation of the preparation process must be established. This should include the key facts of the prepared formula such as batch number of formula, preparation staff, preparation time, preparation amount and storage temperatures. A retention sample of each prepared batch has to be kept for at least 5 days, preferably deep frozen.

Cleaning and disinfections:

- The cleaning process has to be validated for the different materials in use (glass, polycarbonate, etc.) for the temperature applied, detergents and disinfectants, the application times and the used disinfection equipment.

- Hygiene monitoring in the milk preparation room:

- The milk preparation room must be part of the general environmental monitoring of the hospital. Microbiological surface swabs have to be taken from critical spots. General hygiene parameters such as total plate count should be included as well as critical parameters such as *Salmonella, Cronobacter* and *Enterobacteriaceae*.

Requirements for personnel:

- The personal hygiene of the employed staff has to be defined according to hand washing and disinfection. The hand washing and disinfection should be monitored by microbiological hand swabs on regular basis. Jewellery, skin piercings artificial fingernails and nail polish are not accepted. Behaviour rules for the milk preparation room have to be defined e.g. the use of cell phones is not allowed and people with gastric or respiratory infections are not allowed in the room. The work clothing has to be worn exclusively in the milk preparation room. Hair and beards have to be covered and for critical operations, a mouth mask and possibly disposable gloves should be worn.

Quality controls (microbiological monitoring):

- The prepared formula, extracted human milk and the used materials like powders and equipment should be monitored on a regular basis. Details on the quality parameters of infant formula have been described before.

## 6. Conclusions

The personnel employed in the milk preparation room must have the appropriate qualifications to ensure compliance with these special hygienic requirements. The in-house monitoring systems and hygiene management measures have to be the subject of regular instructions and training. Personal hygiene, like regular, hygienic hand washing, and wearing of hygienic clothing, including a head covering and possibly disposable gloves, is the personal responsibility of each employee. The hygienic approach to infant formula preparation and compliance with all guidelines, together with the full documentation and reporting of deviations from these rules is a management task for the concerned section.

In the case of premature babies and immunocompromised infants, the assessment of the individual nutritional requirements is the responsibility of the medical practitioner. This includes also the risk assessment for lactogenic viruses. There are some viruses, which can be transferred from the lactating mother to the newborn with human milk. The risks of infection have to be assessed individually regarding the clinical situation of the mother and the newborn [71].

In cases where breastmilk is not available sterile ready-to-feed formula products are the best alternative from a hygienic point of view. However, often these formulae do not meet the individual nutritional needs of an especially susceptible group of infants to the fullest extent. Accordingly, these products or the breastmilk must often be enriched with food supplements like breastmilk fortifiers. Their addition poses a hygiene risk and has to be done as hygienically as possible immediately before use as described above.

Powdered infant formula provides some more flexibility to combine the feed according to the individual requirements of the infant. However, the powders are not sterile. The reconstitution of the formula with water at temperatures above 70°C has often been recommended to reduce the microbiological risk. But the procedure has been found to be very inefficient for this purpose. Therefore, a case-by-case decision should be made weighing the potentially damaging effects of heat on the individually formulated nutrient concentrate against the benefits of reducing microbiological risks.

*DOI: http://dx.doi.org/10.5772/intechopen.107861*

## Author details

Matthias Fischer* and Anja Buschulte
Department Biological Safety, German Federal Institute for Risk Assessment, Berlin, Germany

*Address all correspondence to: matthias.fischer@bfr.bund.de

## References

[1] Neal-Kluever A, Fisher J, Grylack J, Kakiuchi-Kiyota S, Halpern W. Physiology of the neonatal gastrointestinal system relevant to the disposition of orally administered medications. Drug Metabolism and Disposition. 2019;**47**(3):296-313

[2] Weaver LT, Laker MF, Nelson R. Intestinal permeability in the newborn. Archives of Disease in Childhood. 1984;**59**(3):236-241

[3] Hacker J, Heesemann J, editors. Molekulare Infektionsbiologie. 1st ed. Heidelberg, Berlin Spektrum: Akademischer Verlag; 2000

[4] Willyard C. Could baby's first bacteria take root before birth? Nature. 2018;**553**(7688):264-266

[5] El Edelbi RA, Lindemalm S, Nydert P, Eksborg S. Estimation of body surface area in neonates, infants, and children using body weight alone. International Journal of Pediatrics and Adolescent Medicine. 2021;**8**(4):221-228

[6] Millar M, Wilks M, Costeloe K. Probiotics for preterm infants? Archives of Disease in Childhood. Fetal and Neonatal Edition. 2003;**88**(5):F354-F358

[7] Athalye-Jape G, Patole S. Probiotics for preterm infants – Time to end all controversies. Microbial Biotechnology. 2019;**12**(2):249-253

[8] Al Faleh K, Anabrees J, Bassler D, Al-Kharfi T. Probiotics for prevention of necrotizing enterocolitis in preterm infants. Cochrane Database of Systematic Reviews. 2011;**16**(3):CD005496

[9] D'Agostin M, Squillaci D, Lazzerini M, Barbi E, Lotte Wijers L, Da Lozzo P. Invasive infections associated with the use of probiotics in children: A systematic review. Children. 2021;**8**(10):924

[10] Bertelli C, Pillonel T, Torregrossa A, Prod'hom G, Fischer CJ, Greub G, et al. Bifidobacterium longum bacteremia in preterm infants receiving probiotics. Clinical Infectious Diseases. 2015;**60**(6):924-927

[11] Esaiassen E, Cavanagh P, Hjerde E, Simonsen GS, Støen R, Klingenberg C. Bifidobacterium longum subspecies infantis bacteremia in 3 extremely preterm infants receiving probiotics. Emerging Infectious Diseases. 2016;**22**(9):1664-1666

[12] Vallabhaneni S, Walker TA, Lockhart SR, Ng D, Chiller T, Melchreit R, et al. Fatal gastrointestinal Mucormycosis in a premature infant associated with a contaminated dietary supplement — Connecticut, 2014. MMWR. 2015;**64**(6):155-156

[13] Fleischer-Michaelsen K, Weaver L, Branca F, Robertson A. Feeding and Nutrition of Infants and Young Children. Copenhagen: WHO Regional Publications European Series; 2003

[14] FAO/WHO. *Enterobacter sakazakii* and *Salmonella* in powdered infant formula. Meeting Report. Joint FAO/WHO Technical Meeting on *Enterobacter sakazakii* and *Salmonella* powdered infant formula. Rome, Italy 16-20 Jan 06. FAO/WHO, Microbiological Risk Assessment. 2006

[15] Minor LL. Genus *Salmonella*. In: Sneath PHA, Mair MS, Sharpe ME, Holt JG, editors. Bergey's Manual of Systematic Bacteriology. Vol. 1.

Baltimore: Williams and Wilkins; 1986. pp. 427-458

[16] Doyle MP, editor. Foodborne Bacterial Pathogens. New York/Basel: Marcel Dekker Inc.; 1989. pp. 328-412

[17] Palla MR, Harohalli S, Crawford TN, Desai N. Progression of gastric acid production in preterm neonates: Utilization of In-vitro method. Frontiers in Pediatrics. 2018;**7**(6):211

[18] Lee A, de Lencastre H, Garau J, Kluytmans J, Malhotra-Kumar S, Peschel A, et al. Methicillin-resistant *Staphylococcus aureus*. Nature Reviews. Disease Primers. 2018;**4**:18033

[19] Jay JM, Loessner MJ, Golden DA. Modern Food Microbiology. 7th ed. New York: Springer Science and Business Media Inc.; 2005. pp. 619-631

[20] Blaser MJ, Newsman LS. A review of human salmonellosis: I. Infective dose. Diseases. 1982;**4**(6):1096-1106

[21] Iversen C, Lehner A, Mullane N, Bidlas E, Cleenwerck I, Marugg J, et al. The taxonomy of Enterobacter sakazakii: Proposal of a new genus *Cronobacter* gen. Nov. and descriptions of Cronobacter sakazakii comb. nov. *Cronobacter sakazakii* subsp. *sakazakii*, comb. nov., *Cronobacter sakazakii* subsp. *malonaticus* subsp. nov., *Cronobacter turicensis* sp. nov., *Cronobacter muytjensii* sp. nov., *Cronobacter dublinensis* sp. nov. and *Cronobacter genomospecies* 1. BMC Evolutionary Biology. 2007;**17**(7):64

[22] Nazarowec-White M, Farber JM. Incidence survival and growth of *Enterobacter sakazakii* in infant formula. Journal of Food Protection. 1997;**60**(3):226-230

[23] Iversen C, Lane M, Forsythe SJ. The growth profile, thermotolerance and biofilm formation of *Enterobacter sakazakii* grown in infant formula milk. Letters in Applied Microbiology. 2004;**38**(5):378-382

[24] Arku B, Mullane N, Fox E, Fanning S, Jordan K. *Enterobacter sakazakii* survives spray drying. International Journal of Dairy Technology. 2008;**61**(1):102-108

[25] Edelson-Mammel SG, Porteous MK, Buchanan RL. Survival of *Enterobacter sakazakii* in a dehydrated powdered infant formula. Journal of Food Protection. 2005;**68**(9):1900-1902

[26] Jaradat ZW, Ababneh QO, Saadoun IM, Samara NA, Rashdan AM. Isolation of *Cronobacter* spp. (formerly *Enterobacter sakazakii*) from infant food, herbs and environmental samples and the subsequent identification and confirmation of the isolates using biochemical, chromogenic assays, PCR and 16S rRNA sequencing. BMC Microbiology. 2009;**27**(9):225

[27] Kandhai MC, Reij MW, Gorris LG, Guillaume-Gentil O, van Schothorst M. Occurrence of *Enterobacter sakazakii* in food production environments and households. Lancet. 2004;**363**(9402):39-40

[28] Schmid M, Iversen C, Gontia I, Stephan R, Hofmann A, Hartmann A, et al. Evidence for a plant-associated natural habitat for *Cronobacter* spp. Research in Microbiology. 2009;**160**(8):608-614

[29] Forsythe SJ. Updates on the *Cronobacter* genus. Annual Review of Food Science and Technology. 2018;**25**(9):23-44

[30] Henry M, Fouladkhah A. Outbreak history, biofilm formation, and preventive measures for control of *Cronobacter sakazakii* in infant formula

and infant care settings. Microorganisms. 2019;**7**(3):77

[31] Strysko J, Cope JR, Martin H, Tarr C, Hise K, Collier S, et al. Food safety and invasive *Cronobacter* infections during early infancy, 1961-2018. Emerging Infectious Diseases. 2020;**26**(5):857-865

[32] AFSSA. Descriptive datasheet of microbials transmissible by foodstuff: Enterobacter sakazakii. [Internet]. 2006. Available from: http://www.infectiologie.com/site/medias/_documents/officiels/afssa/Esakazakii090207.pdf [Accessed: August 02, 2022]

[33] Friedemann M. *Enterobacter sakazakii* in powdered infant formula. Bundesgesundheitsblatt, Gesundheitsforschung, Gesundheitsschutz. 2008;**51**(6):664-674

[34] van Acker J, de Smet F, Muyldermans G, Bougatef A, Naessens A, Lauwers S. Outbreak of necrotizing enterocolitis associated with *Enterobacter sakazakii* in powdered milk formula. Journal of Clinical Microbiology. 2001;**39**(1):293-297

[35] Blackshaw K, Valtchev P, Koolaji N, Berry N, Schindeler A, Dehghani F, et al. The risk of infectious pathogens in breast-feeding, donated human milk and breast milk substitutes. Public Health Nutrition. 2020;**24**(7):1725-1740

[36] Hurrell E, Kucerova E, Loughlin M, Caubilla-Barron J, Hilton A, Armstrong R. Neonatal enteral feeding tubes as loci for colonisation by members of the *Enterobacteriaceae*. BMC Infectious Diseases. 2009;**1**(9):146

[37] Stojanović MM, Katić V, Kuzmanović J. Isolation of *Cronobacter sakazakii* from different herbal teas. Vojnosanitetski Pregled. 2011;**68**(10):837-841

[38] Akduman G, Korkmaz IO. Microbial evaluation of turkish herbal teas before and after infusion. Journal of Food Quality and Hazards Control. 2020;**7**:170-174

[39] Daschner FD, Ruden H, Simon R, Clotten J. Microbiological contamination of drinking water in a commercial household water filter system. European Journal of Clinical Microbiology & Infectious Diseases. 1996;**15**(3):233-237

[40] Wilson C, Dettenkofer M, Jonas D, Daschner FD. Pathogen growth in herbal teas used in clinical settings: A possible source of nosocomial infection? American Journal of Infection Control. 2004;**32**(2):117-119

[41] The United States Pharmacopeial Convention FAQs. Chapter 62 Microbial Enumeration of Nonsterile Products: Tests for Specified Microorganisms. [Internet]. 2022. Available from: https://www.usp.org/frequently-asked-questions/microbial-enumeration-nonsterile-products-tests-specified-microorganisms [Accessed: July 14, 2022]

[42] Neill MA, Tarr PI, Taylor DN, Wolf M. Escherichia coli. In: Hui YH, Pierson MD, Gorham JR, editors. Foodborne Disease Handbook: Diseases Caused by Bacteria. 2nd ed. New York: Marcel Dekker; 2001. pp. 169-212

[43] Wang H, Qi J, Dong Y, Li Y, Xu X, Zhou G. Characterization of attachment and biofilm formation by meat-borne E*nterobacteriaceae* strains associated with spoilage. LWT - Food Science and Technology. 2017;**86**:399-407

[44] Ramos-Vivas J, Chapartegui-González I, Fernández-Martínez M, González-Rico C, Fortún J, Escudero R, et al. Biofilm formation by multidrugresistant *Enterobacteriaceae* strainsisolated from solid organ transplantrecipients. Scientific Reports. 2019;**9**:8928

[45] Halligan A, Lawley R. Micro-Facts, a Working Company for Food Microbiologists. Surrey: Leatherhead Food R.A; 1998

[46] Commission Regulation (EC) No 2073/2005 on microbiological criteria for foodstuffs

[47] FAO/WHO Expert Meeting on *Enterobacter sakazakii* and Other Microorganisms in Powdered Infant Formula. *Enterobacter sakazakii* and other microorganisms in powdered infant formula: Meeting report. Microbiological Risk Assessment Series 2004; No. 6. World Health Organization Food and Agriculture Organization of the United Nations

[48] Becker H, Schaller G, von Wiese W, Terplan G. *Bacillus cereus* in infant foods and dried milk products. International Journal of Food Microbiology. 1994;**23**(1):1-15

[49] Cormontagne D, Rigourd V, Vidic J, Rizzotto F, Bille E, Ramarao N. *Bacillus cereus* induces severe infections in preterm neonates: Implication at the hospital and human Milk Bank level. Toxins. 2021;**13**:123

[50] Lewin A, Quach C, Rigourd V, Picaud JC, Perreault T, Frange P, et al. *Bacillus cereus* infection in neonates and the absence of evidence for the role of banked human milk: Case reports and literature review. Infection Control & Hospital Epidemiology. 2019;**40**:787-793

[51] Shaw AG, Cornwell E, Sim K, Thrower H, Scott H, Brown JCS, et al. Dynamics of toxigenic *Clostridium perfringens* colonisation in a cohort of prematurely born neonatal infants. BMC Pediatrics. 2020;**20**:75

[52] Horowitz BZ. Botulinum Toxin. Critical Care Clinics. 2005;**21**(4):825-839

[53] Lund BM. Foodborne disease due to Bacillus and *Clostridium* species. The Lancet. 1990;**336**(8721):982-986

[54] Brett MM, McLauchlin J, Harris A, O'Brien S, Black N, Forsyth RJ, et al. A case of infant botulinum with a possible link to infant formula milk powder: Evidence for the presence of more than one strain of *Clostridium botulinum* in clinical specimens and food. Journal of Medical Microbiology. 2005;**54**(Pt8):769-776

[55] Johnson EA, Tepp WH, Bradshaw M, Gilbert RJ, Cook PE, McIntosh EDG. Characterization of *Clostridium botulinum* strains associated with an infant botulinum case in the United Kingdom. Journal of Clinical Microbiology. 2005;**43**(6):2602-2607

[56] Farber M, Peterkin PI. *Listeria monocytogenes*, a food-borne pathogen. Microbiological Reviews. 1991;**55**(3):476-511

[57] Okike IO, Lamont RF, Heath PT. Do we really need to worry about *Listeria* in newborn infants? The Pediatric Infectious Disease Journal. 2013;**32**(4):405-406

[58] Jones TF, Kellum ME, Porter SS, Bell M, Schaffner W. An outbreak of community-acquired foodborne illness caused by methicillin-resistant *Staphylococcus aureus*. Emerging Infectious Diseases. 2002;**8**(1):82-84

[59] Lee NC, Chen SJ, Tang RB, Hwang BT. Neonatal bacteremia in a neonatal intensive care unit: Analysis of causative organisms and antimicrobial susceptibility. Journal of the Chinese Medical Association. 2004;**67**(1):15-20

[60] Kaufman D, Fairchild KD. Clinical microbiology of bacterial and fungal sepsis in very-low-birthweight

infants. Clinical Microbiology Review. 2004;**17**(3):638-680

[61] Code of Hygienic Practice for powdered Formulae for infants and young children. CAC/RCP. 2008:66

[62] Code of Federal Regulations Title 21. Food and Drugs chapter I—Food and Drug Administration subchapter B—Food for human consumption part 106. Infant Formula Requirements Pertaining To Current Good Manufacturing Practice, Quality Control Procedures, Quality Factors, Records and Reports, and Notifications. §106.55 Controls to prevent adulteration from microorganisms. 2022

[63] Fischer M, Zhu S, de Ree E. Culture media for the detection of Clostria in food. In: Corry JEL, Curtis GDW, Baird RM, editors. Handbook of Culture Media for Food and Water Microbiology. 3rd ed. Cambridge: RSC Publishing; 2012. pp. 66-89

[64] ICMSF: Usefulness of testing for *Clostridium botulinum* in powdered infant formula and dairy-based ingredients for infant formula. 2014

[65] Eaton TJ, Gasson MJ. Molecular screening of *Enterococcus* virulence determinants and potential for genetic exchange between food and medical isolates. Applied and Environmental Microbiology. 2001;**67**(4):1628-1635

[66] Kang TM, Park JH. Isolation of *Enterococcus* from powdered infant and follow-on formulas, and their antibiotic Susceptibilites. Food Science and Biotechnology. 2012;**21**(4):1113-1118

[67] Rajput IR, Khaskheli M, Rao S, Fazlani SA, Shah QA, Khaskheli GB. Microbial quality of formulated infant Milk powders. Journal of Nutrition. 2009;**8**(10):1665-1670

[68] WHO. Safe preparation, storage and handling of powdered infant formula. [Internet]. 2007. Available from: https://www.who.int/publications/i/item/9789241595414 [Accessed: July 11, 2022]

[69] BfR Opinion: Recommendations for the hygienic preparation of powdered infant formula Updated BfR Opinion no. 009/2022 of 29 March 2022, doi:10.17590/20220510-104706

[70] Burgemeister A, Riegel G, Dreisbach J, Friese B, Hesse B, Lohoff R, et al. (Arbeitsgruppe "Hygiene" der GKinD): Hygienische Anforderungen an die Milchküche. Hygiene Medical. 2006;**31**(6):278-281

[71] Ad-hoc-Arbeitskreis Stillschutz: Hinweise und Empfehlungen zum Schutz stillender Frauen vor einer unverantwortbaren Gefährdung durch Gefahr- und Biostoffe insbesondere im Hinblick auf eine Wirkung auf oder über die Laktation. [Internet]. 2019. Available from: https://rp.baden-wuerttemberg.de/fileadmin/RP-Internet/Themenportal/Wirtschaft/Mutterschutz/Documents/Mutter_Stillschutz.pdf [Accessed: July 15, 2022]

Chapter 3

# About a New Palpation Sign in the Diagnosis of Acute Appendicitis in Children and Women of Childbearing Age

*Vitezslav Marek, Stefan Durdik and Roman Zahorec*


## Abstract

Acute appendicitis (AA) is defined as nonspecific bacterial inflammation of the appendix vermiformis and is the most common acute abdominal condition requiring surgical intervention. The clinical picture of atypical forms of AA (children, women of childbearing age) is often insidious with its unpredictable onset and course. The diagnosis is particularly problematic. The new palpation sign consists of two reflex arcs. The visceral reflex arc ensures the diagnosis of an early stage of acute appendicitis, on the other hand, the somatic reflex arc points to the late stage of acute appendicitis. Due to the technical simplicity of the new palpation sign and the positioning of the patient during the examination, it is effective in a restless and distrustful child, as well as in women of childbearing age in differentiating AA from a gynecological disease.


**Keywords:** new palpation sign, visceral reflex arc, somatic reflex arc, children, women of childbearing age

## 1. Introduction

Almost 140 years after its first description by Fitz (1886), acute appendicitis (AA) remains an insidious, unpredictable, and dangerous disease, which causes diagnostic difficulties with its unpredictable onset and course. The diagnosis of atypical forms of AA is particularly problematic, especially in children and women of childbearing age.

Overall, 1–8% of children presenting with abdominal pain have AA [1]. In young children (newborns and infants), appendicitis is an uncommon event with a varied presentation and complications that can develop rapidly [1]. The incidence of acute appendicitis gradually increases after birth, peaks during the late teens, and gradually declines in the geriatric age. A Danish study reported an annual incidence of 2.22/10,000 among boys under 4 years of age and 1.82/10,000 among girls under 4 years of age. The annual incidence among 10–19-year-old boys and girls was 22/10,000 and 18/10,000, respectively [2]. The rate of incorrect diagnosis concerning AA ranges from 28% to 57% in 2–12-year-old children, and is almost 100% in children under 2 years of age [3]. The risk of AA perforation decreases with the child's



IntechOpen

age as follows: 100% < 1 year; 100% 1–2 years; 83.3% 2–3 years; 71.4% 3–4 years; 78.6% 4–5 years, and 47.3% 5 years [4]. The reason is delayed diagnosis of the disease in young children.

Early diagnosis of AA in children is therefore a challenge for the physicians.

In women of childbearing age, the anatomical proximity of the appendix vermiformis to the internal genitalia causes frequent diagnostic confusion of AA with gynecological diseases (e.g., an ectopic pregnancy, pelvic inflammatory disease, midcycle pain occurring with ovulation, endometriosis, ovarian torsion) [5, 6]. AA is more common in men than in women (3:2) [7]. Despite this statistical data, the risk of a lifelong acute appendectomy in women is higher than in men (2:1), which can be explained by the more difficult diagnosis of AA in women, with a higher number of preventive appendectomies with negative histological findings [7].

In this chapter, we present scientific and medical societies a new palpation sign as a reliable tool for the diagnosis of atypical forms of AA (i.e., in children and women of childbearing age) and an effective indicator for surgical intervention.

## 2. New palpation sign

The new palpation sign (described by Vitezslav Marek in 2020) belongs to the group of viscerosomatic palpation signs. Its benefit lies in the diagnosis of AA in patients at risk, such as children and women of childbearing age.

### 2.1 Description of the new palpation sign

"We place the patient on his/her left side with their knees bent. In children, we palpate the abdomen with our right hand. The thumb is located in the lumbar region and pushes into the abdominal cavity. Using 2–4 fingers, the surgeon pushes the abdominal wall of the right hypogastrium into the abdominal cavity. If we notice pulsation of the iliac artery, the sign is considered negative, i.e., this sign excludes AA. If a deep palpation induces a contracture of the abdominal wall (abdominal guarding) which does not allow the pulsation of the iliac arteries to be felt, even when the child is exhaling, the sign is considered positive, i.e., there is a high probability of acute appendicitis (**Figure 1**)" [8, 9].

"We examine the abdomen of a woman of childbearing age bimanually. The thumbs press on the lumbar region, pushing it into the abdominal cavity. Using the fingers of both hands, the surgeon pushes the abdominal wall of the right hypogastrium into the abdominal cavity. With pulsation of the iliac artery during palpation, the sign is considered negative, i.e., it excludes AA. Attention should be paid to examining the internal genitalia of the woman. If deep palpation induces a contracture of the abdominal wall (abdominal guarding) that does not allow the pulsation of the iliac artery to be felt, the sign is considered positive, i.e., there is high probability of acute appendicitis (**Figure 2**)" [8, 9].

### 2.2 Clinical anatomy of the new palpation sign

Neurological basis of the palpation sign is a combination of a somatomotor and visceromotor segmental reflex mediated by the intercostal nerves (Th6–Th12). Reflexes are activated through deep palpation of the abdominal wall of the right hypogastrium, which touches and compresses the inflamed appendix vermiformis [8].

*DOI: http://dx.doi.org/10.5772/intechopen.108951*

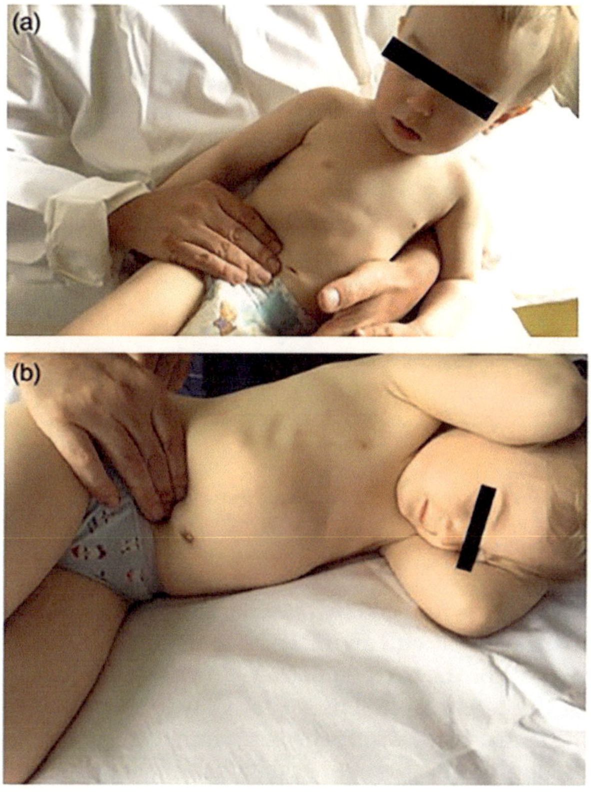


**Figure 1.**
*(a) Examination of a child younger than 3 years of age. Position of the "pietá di Michelangelo" (authors archive).*
*(b) Examination of a child older than 3 years of age (authors archive).*

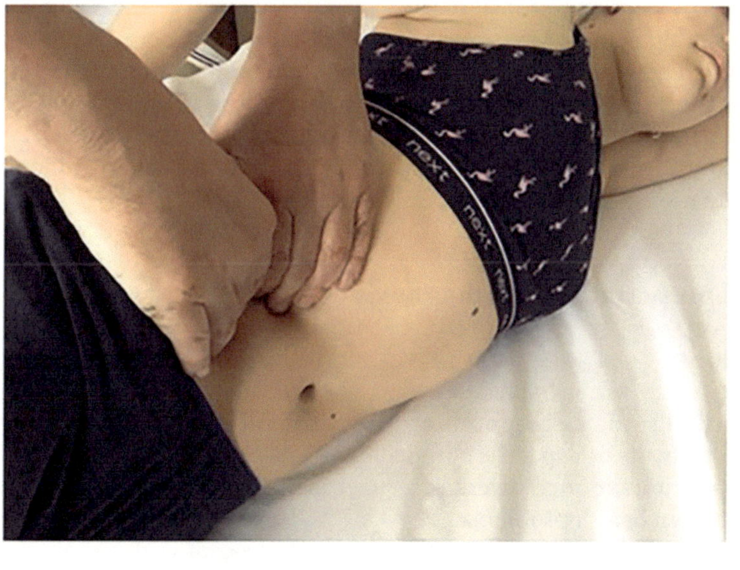


**Figure 2.**
*Examination of a woman of childbearing age (authors archive).*

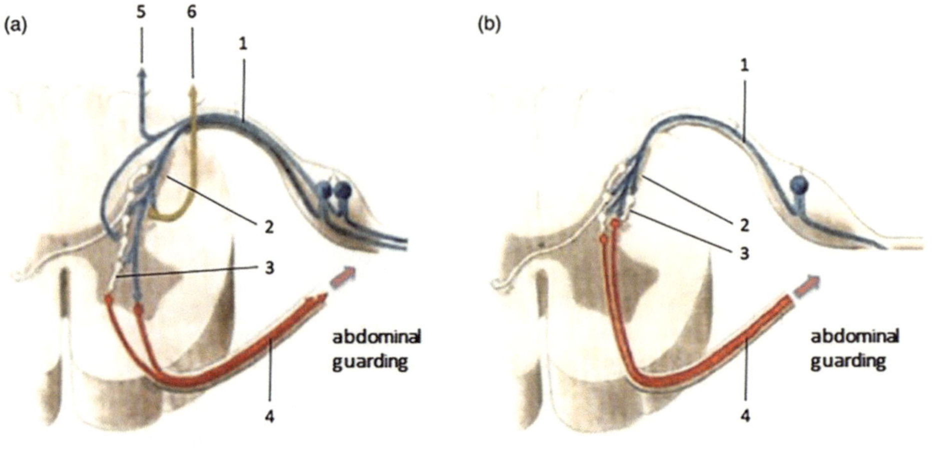


**Figure 3.**
*(a) Somatomotor reflex. (b) Visceromotor reflex. 1, Afferent fibers of the pseudo unipolar cell; 2, posterior spinal roots; 3, interneuron; 4, alpha motor neuron; 5, associated ascending pathways (into the brain); 6, associated ascending pathways (into the brain) [10].*

The somatomotor reflex is induced by pressing the inflamed parietal peritoneum of the abdominal wall of a patient with an inflamed appendix. The nerve impulse is transmitted from the receptors of the parietal peritoneum of the abdominal wall through the afferent fibers of the cerebrospinal nerve pathway to the spinal ganglion cells in the posterior roots of the spinal cord, where they are connected to the alpha motor neuron via an interneuron. The alpha motor neuron originates from the anterior spinal roots, innervates the abdominal muscles, and activates the abdominal guarding [8].

Visceromotor reflex is formed by compression of the inflamed appendix through the abdominal wall, no peritonitis is required. The nerve impulse transmits from receptors located in the appendix wall (the Pacinian bodies and the free nerve endings) through the afferent splanchnic nerve pathway to the posterior roots of the spinal cord. The close anatomical location of afferent splanchnic, cerebrospinal fibers, and the alpha motor neuron causes the intense signal created by compression of the inflamed appendix to induce a "spillover" phenomenon with direct activation of the alpha motor neuron, causing abdominal guarding (**Figure 3**) [8].

Activation of the somatomotor and visceromotor reflex results in spasm of the abdominal muscles—"abdominal guarding"—preventing deeper abdominal palpation and palpation of the iliac artery pulsations [8].

## 3. Clinical presentation and diagnosis of AA

### 3.1 Children

In early childhood, the diagnosis of AA is difficult and in most cases delayed. This delay is caused by its nonspecific clinical manifestation, which is often covered up by other nonspecific childhood diseases, as well as the child's inability to describe and specify their own health problems.

**Newborns (birth to 30 days)** with AA usually present with abdominal distension in 60% to 90%, vomiting 59%, palpable mass 20–40%, irritability or lethargy in 22%,

*DOI: http://dx.doi.org/10.5772/intechopen.108951*

cellulitis of abdominal wall in 12–16%, hypotension, hypothermia, and respiratory distress [11]. AA is rare in this age group. This is explainable by the so-called fetal appendix shape (orificium of the appendix to the caecum is wide) with a low tendency to obstruction of the lumen and subsequent formation of AA.

AA in newborns progresses rapidly due to:

- a small omentum majus—unable to limit inflammation in the right hypogastrium,
- low plasticity of the peritoneum—the inability to isolate and limit inflammation,
- low resistance of the child's organism to infection.

**Infants and toddlers (less than 3 years)** with AA usually do not respond to caressing and are not satisfied in their mother's arms. In most cases, a caring mother only suspects that the child has a stomach ache, but cannot explain it exactly. In such cases, the recommendation of Professor Tosovsky applies: "We must never underestimate and contradict mother's opinion, thinking that our professional knowledge entitles us to do so. It is the quickest way to a mistake" [12]. Maternal instinct is important in diagnosing AA in this age group. It is questionable whether mothers who prioritize career and personal life over child care have developed this maternal bond.

The prominent symptoms in this age group are vomiting (85–90%), pain (35–81%), fever (40–60%), diarrhea (18–46%), cough or rhinitis (40%), grunting respiration (8–23%), right hip mobility restriction, pain, and limping in 3–23% [13].

**Preschool (age 3–5 years).** Even in this age group, the incidence of AA is rare and accounts for less than 5% of all childhood appendicitis [1]. With growing age, children are able to communicate well and can describe the symptoms of acute appendicitis, early diagnosis of acute appendicitis becomes more easy and accurate. Abdominal pain dominates in AA in pre-school children (89–100%). This is followed by vomiting (66–100%), fever (80–87%), and anorexia (53–60%) [1].

#### *3.1.1 Clinical examination*

During the clinical examination of the abdomen, each patient is approached individually.

The nature of the child, the level of dissimulation is assessed through calm and repeated examinations. When palpating the abdomen, the overall reactions of the child are evaluated—facial redness, involuntary movements of the limbs, and

Macenko's interesting observation: "...when palpating in the right hypogastrium, the child pulls the right lower limb and pulls the examiner's hand away" [14].

The effort is to identify palpable pain in the right hypogastrium and the presence of peritoneal irritation, which represents a "sign over sign." A certain degree of experience is necessary to distinguish the protective muscle tension of the abdominal wall (abdominal guarding in peritonitis) from the free contraction of the abdominal wall in children due to their fear. The new palpation sign eliminates this disadvantage. Its essence is the palpation of the pulsation of the iliac artery, not the subjective assessment of pain and reflex tension of the abdominal muscles. Palpation of the pulsation of the iliac arteries is an objective indicator that is not affected by the restlessness of the child.

### *3.1.2 Ultrasonography (US)*

Using US for the acute appendicitis diagnosis is convenient and safe, but its effectiveness is highly operator dependent. Basic ultrasound findings indicating acute appendicitis are: swollen appendix (diameter > 6 mm), an appendicolith, high echogenicity surrounding the appendix (caused by inflammation), pericecal free fluid, and thickened bowel loops with weakened peristalsis [15, 16]. The analysis by Yasmine Lounis et al. found that the sensitivity for first abdominal US diagnosing AA in children was 65.5%. In most of children in whom abdominal ultrasound was false negative, appendix was either not or incompletely visualized [17].

### *3.1.3 Computed tomography (CT), magnetic resonance imaging (MRI)*

CT has been considered the radiological gold standard to confirm clinical and US suspicion of appendicitis with high sensitivity and specificity (72–99% and 84%) [18]. Among the basic diagnostic signs in a CT examination of a child with AA are:

swollen appendix (diameter more than 6 mm), focal apical thickening of the appendix, lymphadenopathy, presence of an appendicolith and abscesses [16]. Repeated CT carries a proven risk of increased cancer incidence in children, and its use should therefore be limited to clear indications with a well-defined risk-benefit ratio [19]. Advantages of CT include less operator dependence, easier visualization of the retrocecal appendix, and less intestinal gas interference.

A Finnish study demonstrated comparable diagnostic accuracy of contrast-enhanced low- dose CT and standard CT in the diagnosis of AA, with the mean radiation dose of low-dose CT significantly reduced (3.33 vs. 4.44 mSv) [20].

Magnetic resonance imaging (MRI) is a feasible alternative to CT for secondary imaging in AA in children and can reliably distinguish perforated from non-perforated AA [21].

### *3.1.4 Biochemical and hematological markers*

Various biochemical and hematological markers have been established for improving the diagnostic accuracy of acute appendicitis in younger children (**Table 1**). Below the common ones are discussed:

### *3.1.5 Complete blood count (CBC) and CRP*

Although the white blood cell (WBC) count is increased in acute appendicitis, still it is nonspecific and insensitive. Furthermore, the WBC count cannot differentiate between a complicated and an uncomplicated acute appendicitis.

C-reactive protein (CRP) is a nonspecific inflammatory mediator. It has a sensitivity of 43–92% and a specificity of 33–95% for diagnosing acute appendicitis in children presenting with abdominal pain [23]. The sensitivity of leukocytosis and increased neutrophil count may approach 98% with an elevated CRP for diagnosing acute appendicitis [24].

### *3.1.6 Neutrophils-to-lymphocytes (NLR) ratio*

The neutrophil-to-lymphocyte ratio (NLR) is a simple, inexpensive, and reliable parameter of systemic inflammation. The NLR is derived from a differential of white blood cells when the number of circulating neutrophils is divided by the number of

| In blood/serum | In urine |
|---|---|
| White blood cell count (WBC) | Urine 5-hydroxyindoleacetic acid (5-HIAA) |
| Differential leukocyte counts (DLC | Urine leucine-rich alpha glycoprotein-2 (LRG) |
| C-reactive proteins (CRP) | |
| Erythrocyte sedimentation reaction (ESR) | |
| Tumor necrosis factor alpha (TNF-alpha), acid) | |
| Alpha1-glycoprotein (alpha1gp) | |
| Leucocyte elastase complex (elastase) | |
| Interleukin-8 (IL-8) | |
| Interleukin-6 (IL-6) | |
| Interleukin-10 ( IL-10) | |
| Granulocyte colony stimulating factor | |
| Interferon gamma | |
| Soluble intercellular adhesion molecule-1 | |
| Matrix metalloproteinase-9 | |
| Tissue inhibitor metalloproteinase-1 | |
| Serum amyloid A | |
| Plasma calprotectin | |
| Plasma serotonin | |
| Serum leucine-rich alpha glycoprotein-2 (LRG) | |
| Procalcitonin | |

**Table 1.**
*The most common biological markers used in the diagnosis of appendicitis [22].*

circulating lymphocytes. Kahramanca et al. reported NLR limit values of 4.68 (65% sensitivity, 55% specificity) for the diagnostics of acute appendicitis and NLR ≥ 5.74 (71% sensitivity, 49% specificity) for distinguishing between complicated and uncomplicated appendicitis [25]. Shashirekha et al. reported NLR limit values of 3.0 (81% sensitivity, 53% specificity) and 5.5 (78.4% sensitivity, 41.7% specificity) for the diagnostics of AA and perforated appendicitis, respectively [26].

A combination of clinical examination (with new palpation sign), laboratory tests, and US may significantly improve diagnostic sensitivity and specificity.

### *3.1.7 Algorithm for diagnosis and treatment of children with suspected AA*

Acute appendectomy is indicated in children with suspected AA with positive clinical examination (new palpation sign) and a positive US, without the needs of a CT scan or MRI. If the clinical examination (new palpation sign) is negative, if US is suspected, conservative treatment (antibiotic therapy) with patient observation (repeated clinical and US examination every 6 hours) is recommended. MRI or diagnostic +/− therapeutic laparoscopy is indicated for failure of conservative treatment (**Figure 4**) [9].

Several studies on this topic have shown no difference in the rate of postoperative complications between children who underwent appendectomy after failure of

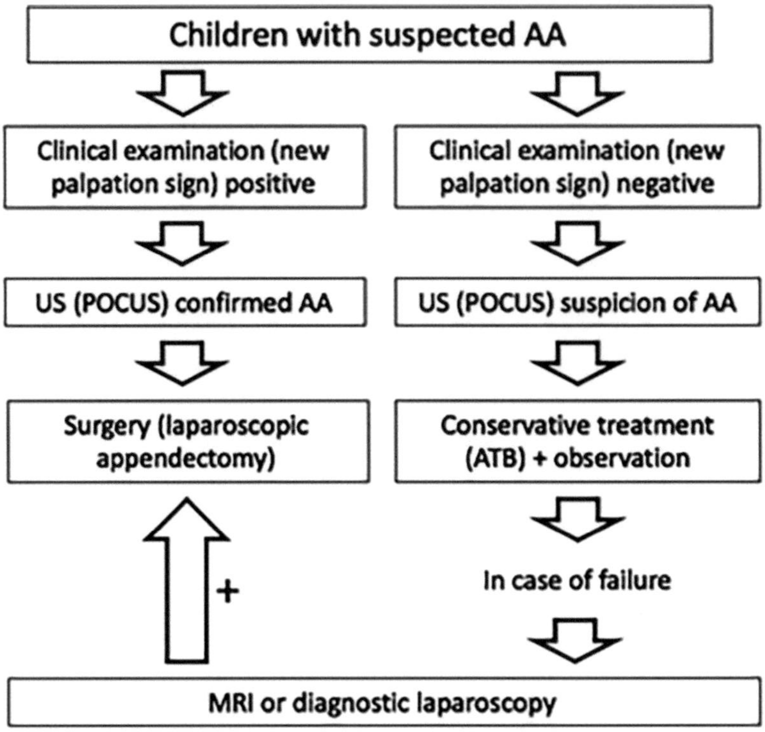


**Figure 4.**
*Algorithm for diagnosis and treatment of children with suspected AA (authors archive).*

conservative (antibiotic) treatment and children who were treated surgically at the first presentation of AA [27, 28].

### 3.2 Women of childbearing age

The course of AA in a woman of childbearing age can be confusing and still presents a diagnostic problem, in which it is necessary to distinguish between gynecological and non-gynecological diseases (**Table 2**).

AA and pelvic inflammatory disease (PID) are two of the most common causes of abdominal pain in women of childbearing age [6]. PID encompasses a spectrum of diseases that include salpingitis, endometritis, and tuboovarian sepsis.

As with AA, the diagnosis of PID is extremely important because more than 60% of women who experience severe PID or multiple episodes of PID become infertile. In addition, missed or delayed diagnosis is associated with chronic pelvic pain and ectopic pregnancy [29].

The first symptom differentiating AA from PID is the duration of abdominal pain. The pain of acute appendicitis usually lasts 24–36 hours, while the pain of PID can last for weeks or until it is treated and is characterized by no worsening.

A study by Morishita et al. from 2007 is currently the most relevant in terms of the clinical picture of these two pathologies. In this retrospective study, data from 181 women with abdominal pain, 109 with a diagnosis of appendicitis, and 72 with PID were analyzed. Women with PID were younger, with bilateral pelvic pain and fever. Conversely, women with acute appendicitis initially had periumbilical pain migrating to the right iliac fossa, loss of appetite, nausea, and vomiting [30].

| **Lower quadrant abdominal pain in young women** | |
|---|---|
| **Non-gynaecological disease** | **Gynaecological disease** |
| Appendicitis | Ectopic pregnancy |
| Crohn's disease | Ruptured follicular or corpus luteum cyst |
| Meckel's diverticulitis | Ovarian torsion |
| Sigmoid diverticulitis | PID |
| Perforated peptic ulcer | Haemorhage of an ovarian cyst |
| Viral gastroenteritis | Mittelschmera |
| Mesenteric adenitis | Endometriosis |
| Ventral and inguinal hernias | |
| Urological disease: | |
| Pyelonephritis | |
| Perinephric abscess | |
| Urolithiasis | |
| Urinary tract infections | |

**Table 2.**
*Differential diagnosis of diseases causing pain in the right hypogastrium in women of childbearing age.*

### *3.2.1 Clinical examination*

During the clinical examination of the abdomen in a woman of childbearing age, the position of the patient at the new palpation sign is used to distinguish AA from PID. Its principle lies in the different degree of fixation of the appendix and internal genitalia in the female abdominal cavity. When positioning the patient with PID on the left side, the maximum palpable pain shifts from the Mc Burney point toward the left hypogastrium, the pulsation of the iliac artery is palpated. On the contrary, in AA, the pain remains fixed at McBurney's point, palpation causes contracture of the abdominal wall and does not allow to feel the pulsation of the iliac arteries.

A complete clinical examination must always include a gynecological examination with a smear from the cervix to detect possible infections and a transvaginal US. In addition, an adequate sexual history should always be investigated (e.g., the presence of an intrauterine device that can cause PID).

### *3.2.2 Ultrasonography (US)*

Among radiological examinations, US is certainly the first diagnostic step in young women of childbearing age with acute abdominal pain. Its sensitivity and specificity are relatively low, because both clinical diagnoses (AA, PID) have similar US sings. Among the US signs defining acute appendicitis can be included: non-compressible, aperistaltic tubular structure with a blind end with a diameter greater than 6 mm, echogenic periappendicular fat (due to inflammation) and hyperemia in the thickened wall of the appendix identified by color Doppler ultrasound [31]. Abdominal ultrasound in the diagnosis of acute appendicitis has a sensitivity of 75–90% and a specificity of 85–98% [16]. In case of an ambiguous diagnosis, transvaginal US is indicated, which enables more accurate visualization of the adnexa and uterus.

### *3.2.3 Computed tomography (CT), magnetic resonance imaging (MRI)*

When the clinical presentation is nonspecific and the ultrasound is non-diagnostic, patients undergo abdominopelvic computer tomography (CT) with contrast medium [30].

Hentour's criteria (appendiceal diameter and left tubal thickening) are used for CT differential diagnosis of AA and PID.

When interpreting an abdominopelvic CT in women of childbearing age with suspected AA, the following procedure is recommended:

1. Measurement of the diameter of the appendix

2. Measurement of the thickness of the left Fallopian tube.

If the diameter of the appendix is < 7 mm and the thickness of the left Fallopian tube ≥ 10 mm, appendicitis is improbable, PID highly probable. If the diameter of the appendix is ≥ 7 mm and the thickness of the Fallopian tube does not reach 10 mm, the diagnosis of AA is confirmed [32]. The most common direct CT signs of PID include:

haziness of the pelvic fat, obscuration of the pelvic fascial planes, thickening of the uterosacral ligaments, abnormal endometrial enhancement with fluid in the endometrial cavity, enhancement and thickening of the fallopian tubes, and enlarged, reactively altered polycystic ovaries [33].

The sensitivity of CT in appendicitis is from 87% to 98%, higher than US [30].

Magnetic resonance plays a secondary role due to its financial complexity. Its advantage is the absence of radiation exposure and excellent specificity and sensitivity in the diagnosis of acute appendicitis or PID. However, it should be reserved for specific population groups (pregnant women, children) [34]. MRI has sensitivity and specificity for diagnosis of appendicitis of 95% and 89%, respectively.

### *3.2.4 Biochemical and hematological markers*

Routine laboratory tests for the diagnosis of AA in women of childbearing age include:

- *Complete blood count, leukocyte count, CRP and NLR.* These are nonspecific indicators of inflammation with low differential diagnostic specificity between AA and PID.

- *Physical and chemical examination of urine* is indicated for the exclusion of urological diseases—kidney or bladder stones (hematuria) or inflammatory diseases of the urinary tract (pyuria, bacteriuria).

- *Biochemical examination of blood with a focus on hepatic tests and serum amylases* is helpful in differentiating diseases of the hepatobiliary tract and pancreas from AA.

- *Examination of human chorionic gonadotropin test (b-hcg)* to exclude an unrecognized or ectopic pregnancy [35].

Second-level laboratory tests may be useful in patients with nonspecific abdominal symptoms. Among them, cervical smear to diagnose genital infections (such as Neisseria

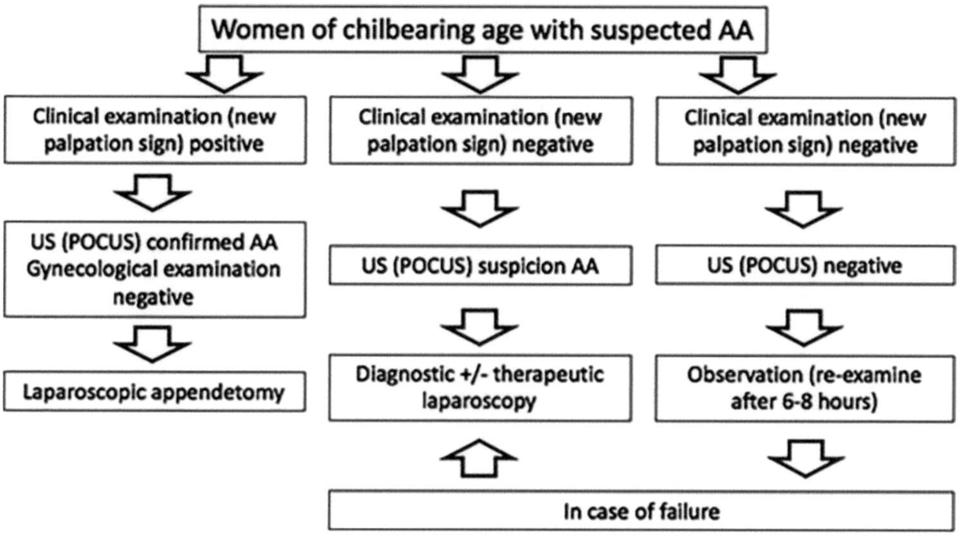


**Figure 5.**
*Algorithm for diagnosis and treatment of women of childbearing age with suspected AA (authors archive).*

gonorrhea or Chlamydia trachomatis) is certainly important, which would support the diagnosis of PID [34]. Rapid tests for the detection of these microorganisms are available. The findings of 10 or more polymorphonuclear (PMN) leukocytes on a gram-stained endocervical smear are diagnostic of mucopurulent cervicitis and may also help confirm the diagnosis of PID [36].

#### *3.2.5 Algorithm for diagnosis and treatment of women of childbearing age with suspected AA*

Laparoscopic appendectomy is indicated in women of childbearing age with suspected AA with positive clinical examination (new palpable sign), high suspicion on US, and negative gynecological examination. If the clinical examination (new palpation symptom) is negative, with high US suspicion, diagnostic +/− therapeutic laparoscopy is recommended (**Figure 5**).

## 4. Conclusion

Despite the intensive technological development of imaging examinations, the medical history and clinical examination of the abdomen in AA remains a basic diagnostic tool.

We introduced a new palpable sign and described its clinical anatomy consisting of two reflex arcs. The visceral reflex arc ensures the diagnosis of the early stage of acute appendicitis. It is activated by compression of the inflamed appendix, no peritonitis is required. Conversely, the somatic reflex arc is activated when the peritoneum is affected by inflammation and indicates the late stage of acute appendicitis.

The examination itself using the new palpation sign is not technically demanding. It can be performed even with a restless and distrustful child. In women of childbearing age, the very position of the patient with a new palpation sign makes it possible to distinguish between gynecological and non-gynecological diseases.

The new palpation sign serves as a reliable indicator for surgery, minimizes unindicated revisions of the abdominal cavity, and is suitable for diagnosing AA in atypical forms (i.e., in children and women of childbearing age) with a sensitivity of 95.57% and a specificity of 95.78% [9].

Due to its material and technical simplicity, it can be used in various parts of the world and in emergency situations where diagnostic equipment and technologies are limited. It represents a first-line diagnostic tool, but also a suitable part of a scoring diagnostic system.

The combination of expertise, experience, and humility of the surgeon turns the diagnosis of AA into a surgical art.

## Acknowledgements

This chapter is dedicated to the children who perished during senseless wars caused by human hatred.

## Author details

Vitezslav Marek[1*], Stefan Durdik[1] and Roman Zahorec[2]

1 Department of Surgical Oncology, St. Elizabeth Hospital, Medical School of Comenius University, Bratislava, Slovak Republic

2 Department of Anestesiology and Intensive Medicine, Medical School of Comenius University, Bratislava, Slovak Republic

*Address all correspondence to: vitezslav.marek@gmail.com

## References

[1] Rothrock SG, Pagane J. Acute appendicitis in children: Emergency department diagnosis and management. Annals of Emergency Medicine. 2000;**36**:39-51

[2] Andersen SB, Paerregaard A, Larsen K. Changes in the epidemiology of acute appendicitis and appendectomy in Danish children 1996-2004. European Journal of Pediatric Surgery. 2009;**19**:286-289

[3] Nance M, Adamson WT, Hedrick HL. Appendicitis in the young child: A continuing diagnostic challenge. Pediatric Emergency Care. 2000;**16**:160-162

[4] Pogorelic Z, Domjanovic J, Jukic M, et al. Acute appendicitis in children younger than five years of age: Diagnostic challenge for pediatric surgeons. Surgical Infections. 2019;**21**:239

[5] Prystowsky JB, Pugh CM, Nagle AP. Appendicitis. Current Problems in Surgery. 2005;**42**:694-742

[6] Kreisel K et al. Prevalence of pelvic inflammatory disease in sexually experienced women of reproductive age-United States, 2013-2014. Annals of Emergency Medicine. 2017;**70**(1):28-30

[7] Brown TW, McCarthy ML, Kelen GD, et al. An epidemiologic study of closed emergency department malpractice claims in a national database of physician malpractice insurers. Academic Emergency Medicine. 2010;**17**:553-560

[8] Marek V, Zahorec R, Durdik S. Acute appendicitis: Clinical anatomy of the new palpation sign. Clinical Anatomy. 2021;**34**(2):1-6

[9] Marek V, Zahorec R, Durdik S. A new palpation sign for the diagnosis of atypical forms of acute appendicitis (children and women of childbearing age). The Journal of Surgical Research. 2022;**5**:101-114

[10] Čihák R. Anatomy 3. Praha, CZ: Grada Press; 1997

[11] Jancelewicz T, Kim G, Miniati D. Neonatal appendicitis: A new look at an old zebra. Journal of Pediatric Surgery. 2008;**43**:e1-e5

[12] Tošovsky VV. Náhle Příhody Břišní u dětí Včasná Diagnostika. Praha: Grada Publishing; 1996. pp. 51-64

[13] Chang Y-T, Lin J-Y, Huang Y-S. Appendicitis in children younger than 3 years of age: An 18-year experience. The Kaohsiung Journal of Medical Sciences. 2006;**22**:432-436

[14] Marek V et al. Akútna apendicitída-včasná diagnostika a predoperačná rozvaha. Praha: Grada Publishing; 2021. p. 117

[15] Puylaert JB. Acute appendicitis: US evaluation using graded compression. Radiology. 1986;**158**:355-360

[16] Vandermeermd FQ, You W, Cheong JJ. Imaging of acute pelvic pain. Topics in Magnetic Resonance Imaging. 2010;**21**(4):201-211

[17] Lounis Y, Hugo J, Demarche M. Influence of age on clinical presentation, diagnosis delay and outcome in pre-school children with acute appendicitis. BMC Pediatrics. 2020;**20**:151

[18] Chang ST, Jeffrey RB, Olcott EW. Three- step sequential positioning algorithm during sonographic evaluation for appendicitis increases appendiceal

visualization rate and reduces CT use. American Journal of Roentgenology. 2014;**203**:1006-1012

[19] Doria AS, Moineddin R, Kellenberger CJ, Epelman M, Beyene J, Schuh S, et al. US or CT for diagnosis of appendicitis in children and adults a meta-analysis. Radiology. 2006;**241**:83-94

[20] Sippola S, Virtanen J, Tammilehto V. The accuracy of low-dose computed tomography protocol in patients with suspected acute appendicitis: The OPTICAP study. Annals of Surgery. 2020;**271**(2):332-338

[21] Rosenbaum DG, Askin G, Beneck DM, et al. Differentiating perforated from non- perforated appendicitis on contrast-enhanced magnetic resonance imaging. Pediatric Radiology. 2017;**47**:1483-1490

[22] Almaramhy HH. Acute appendicitis in young children less than 5 years: review article. Italian Journal of Pediatrics. 2017;**43**:15

[23] Yang HR, Wang YC, Chung PK, Chen WK, Jeng LB, Chen RJ. Role of leukocyte count, neutrophil percentage, and C-reactive protein in the diagnosis of acute appendicitis in the elderly. The American Surgeon. 2005;**71**:344-347

[24] Yu CW, Juan LI, Wu MH, Shen CJ, Wu JY, Lee CC. Systematic review and meta-analysis of the diagnostic accuracy of procalcitonin, C-reactive protein and white blood cell count for suspected acute appendicitis. The British Journal of Surgery. 2013;**100**:322-329

[25] Kahramanca Ş et al. Neutrophil-to-lymphocyte ratio as a predictor of acute appendicitis. Ulus Travma Acil Cerrahi Derg (Turkish Journal of Trauma and Emergency Surgery). 2014;**20**:19-22

[26] Shashirekha CA, Singh R. Sanganboina S, Preoperative neutrophil-to-lymphocyte ratio in predicting the severity of appendicitis: A retrospective cohort study in a tertiary rural hospital. International Journal of Surgery. 2017;**1**:3-6

[27] Svensson JF, Patkova B, Almstrom M, et al. Nonoperative treatment with antibiotics versus surgery for acute nonperforated appendicitis in children: A pilot randomized controlled trial. Annals of Surgery. 2015;**261**:67-71

[28] Minneci PC, Mahida JB, Lodwick DL, et al. Effectiveness of patient choice in nonoperative vs surgical management of pediatric uncomplicated acute appendicitis. JAMA Surgery. 2016;**151**: 408-415

[29] Weström L. Incidence, prevalence, and trends of acute pelvic inflammatory disease and its consequences in industrialized countries. American Journal of Obstetrics and Gynecology. 1980;**138**(7):880-892

[30] Morishita K, Gushimiyagi M, Hashiguchi M, Stein GH, Tokuda Y. Clinical prediction rule to distinguish pelvic inflammatory disease from acute appendicitis in women of childbearing age. The American Journal of Emergency Medicine. 2007;**25**(2):152-157

[31] Molander MVP, Paavonen J, Sjöberg J, Savelli L, Cacciatore B. Transvaginal sonography in the diagnosis of acute appendicitis. Ultrasound in Obstetrics & Gynecology. 2002;**20**(5):496-501

[32] Hentour KE et al. How to differentiate acute pelvic inflammatory disease from acute appendicitis. A decision tree based on CT findings. European Radiology. 2018;**28**(2):673-682

[33] Revzin MV, Mathur M, Dave HB, Macer ML, Spektor M. Pelvic inflammatory disease: Multimodality imaging approach with clinical-pathologic correlation. Radiographics. 2016;**36**(5):1579-1596

[34] Gennaro P et al. Acute abdomen in woman of childbearing age: Appendicitis or pelvic inflammatory disease? A systematic review. Biomedical Journal of Scientific & Technical Research. 2021;**35**(4):27900-27906

[35] Dahlberg DL, Lee C, Fenlon T, Willoughby D. Differential diagnosis of abdominal pain in women of childbearing age. Appendicitis or pelvic inflammatory. Advance for Nurse Practitioners. 2004;**12**(1):40-45

[36] Kruszka P, Kruszka SJ. Evaluation of acute pelvic pain in women. American Family Physician. 2021;**82**(2):141-147

Chapter 4

# Influence of Maternal Exercise on Maternal and Offspring Metabolic Outcomes

*Filip Jevtovic and Linda May*


## Abstract

Epigenetic transmission of metabolic disease to an offspring increases their risk for development of metabolic disease later in life. With the increasing rates of obesity in women of child-bearing age it is critical to develop strategies to prevent perpetuating metabolic disease across generations. Maternal exercise during gestation imprints offspring metabolic phenotype, thus increasing their imperviousness to metabolic assaults later in life. In rodent models, maternal exercise before and during gestation leads to enhanced offspring glycemic control, mitochondrial bioenergetics, and lower adiposity, which decreases their risk for development of future metabolic disease. In humans, maternal gestational exercise decreases pregnancy complications and improves maternal and offspring metabolism on both the whole-body and the cellular level. Maternal exercise restores the obesity-induced metabolic derangements, restoring maternal and offspring metabolic phenotype. While unknown, different exercise modalities might have a differential effect, however, evidence remains scarce.


**Keywords:** pregnancy, prenatal, exercise, fetal, metabolism

## 1. Introduction

Rates of pediatric obesity are escalating worldwide. Increasing rates of childhood obesity are likely to translate into a high cumulative incidence of metabolic disease (i.e., type 2 diabetes mellitus (T2D)) and further exacerbate the strain on the healthcare system, public health, and global economy [1]. The development of obesity is often attributed to a combination of genetic and acquired environmental factors. It is well established that the epigenetic transmission of metabolic diseases to offspring will increase their risk for the development of metabolic disorders later in life [2]. Accordingly, environmental exposures (i.e., overnutrition) experienced by parents during intrauterine and early postnatal life will have profound effects on offspring health. Because of the increasing rates of obesity among individuals of child-bearing age, it is critical to develop strategies to prevent the transgenerational propagation of metabolic disease.

It is widely understood that physical activity induces an array of positive metabolic changes that can delay and/or reverse the deleterious effects of obesity. While the mechanisms of action behind the benefits of regular physical exercise are well-documented, research has mostly focused on the person performing the exercise. Consequently, there is limited understanding in the mechanisms by which regular maternal exercise influences the metabolic phenotype of offspring. Further, while studies regarding the effects of maternal exercise on pregnancy, maternal, and offspring outcomes are available and reviewed [3–8], data which characterizes the mediating factors affecting offspring developmental programming is limited [9]. This is partly due to limitations in revealing the cellular and molecular mechanisms behind maternal exercise-derived benefits that stem from the inability to obtain neonate tissue samples (i.e., skeletal muscle (SkM)).

An understanding of the explicit alterations that maternal exercise causes in the offspring phenotype would allow for the characterization of novel targets and could be used to render different therapeutics for metabolic diseases. Further, elucidating the specific biological mechanisms induced by different exercise modalities could permit this lifestyle intervention to serve analogous to a targeted therapy. Thus, there is potential for different exercise modalities to be used in a prescription-like manner to generate a unique set of metabolic adaptations suitable for treating and/or reducing offspring predispositions to metabolic disease. In view of this possibility, the focus of this chapter will be on describing the mechanisms behind the effects of the maternal exercise on offspring metabolic programing. Emphasis will be on the analysis of the biological mechanisms behind specific metabolic adaptations that promote imperviousness to metabolic challenges (i.e., overnutrition) leading to obesity and T2D. Further, considering that mitochondrial dysfunction and insulin resistance (IR) are major constituents of these metabolic diseases, a focus will be on the alterations in offspring mitochondrial bioenergetics and glycemic control.

## 2. Learning from rodent models

### 2.1 Maternal obesity and offspring health

The use of rodent models has allowed researchers to study how various environmental factors during critical windows of prenatal and early postnatal development alter metabolic phenotype and elicit tissue specific adaptations in progeny. Considering the ever-increasing rates of obesity, dietary habits, particularly overnutrition, during gestation have a critical role in fetal development and are often the focus of investigations. Maternal obesity and often concomitant IR increase the propensity of the development and transmission of metabolic disease onto progeny. A maternal obesogenic diet during fetal life readily programs first and second generation offspring into a T2D-like phenotype, even without additional dietary insults (i.e., overnutrition) administered to these generations [10].

Maternal obesity elicits multifaceted effects on offspring behavioral habits and physiology. Offspring from obese mothers have a tendency to be physically inactive and hyperphagic [11, 12]. Further, offspring adopt a metabolic syndrome-like phenotype with impaired glucose tolerance, higher blood triglycerides, cholesterol, and leptin, but lower adiponectin levels, which increases offspring predisposition for the development of cardiometabolic disease later in life [11, 12]. Maternal obesogenic diet consumption during gestation increases offspring adiposity primarily through adipocyte hypertrophy [12–14]. Adipocyte hypertrophy, rather than hyperplasia, is associated with lower insulin responsiveness, inflammation, and an overall dysregulation of systemic energy metabolism [15]. Increased adiposity is further accompanied by a greater intramuscular fat accretion associated with higher PPARγ mRNA expression which could contribute to the development of lipotoxicity-induced SkM IR observed in these offspring [13]. Offspring from obese mothers have a restricted SkM growth potential which subsequently decreases their SkM cross-sectional area [13]. These alterations combined with lower GLUT4 and insulin receptor mRNA expression, as observed in SkM of offspring from obese mothers, attenuates their potential for insulin-stimulated glucose uptake and increase the propensity of offspring to develop hyperglycemia [13]. Considering that SkM is responsible for the majority of postprandial glucose uptake, these alterations have a profound effect on glucose homeostasis and could increase the risk for the development of T2D. Finally, maternal overnutrition leads to the downregulation of pathways associated with mitochondrial oxidation and lowers mitochondrial electron transport protein expression, leading to mitochondrial dysfunction [14].

Together, these alterations can lead to derangements in energy metabolism later in offspring life and increase their proclivity for metabolic disease. In view of this, it is essential to explore the effects of different lifestyle interventions that can alleviate the detrimental effects of maternal obesity on offspring metabolic dysregulation. Regular exercise is known to be protective against metabolic derangements observed in obesity and T2D in mother and offspring. Accordingly, illumination of the effects of maternal exercise on offspring body composition, glycemic control, and mitochondrial functioning will underline mechanistic alterations behind enhanced metabolic phenotype.

### 2.2 Maternal exercise enhances offspring metabolic phenotype

#### *2.2.1 Body composition*

While most studies support the notion that exercise before and during gestation has an effect on offspring body weight (BW), findings are inconsistent [9]. Reports remain divided between maternal exercise causing a decrease [16–20], increase [21, 22], or having no effect on litter [23–25] or pup BW [26–30]. Additionally, these studies remain divided between maternal exercise leading to less weight gain with aging in offspring or having no effect on age-related weight gain. For example, Quiclet and associates found no effect of maternal exercise on male offspring BW at weaning or at 7 months of age; however, in their subsequent study, a decrease in BW was observed at weaning and 3 months of age, despite using the same animal and exercise model [17, 28]. Similarly, despite the use of the same animal species and exercising method across studies, change in BW is inconsistent in male offspring from exercising mothers at ~12 months of age [29, 30]. In addition to BW, discrepancies regarding the effect of maternal exercise on body composition have been observed across studies and offspring gender [16–18, 21, 23–25, 27–29, 31]. Carter et al. [26] reported an increase in lean mass and subsequent decrease in fat mass in males ~12 months of age; however, this was not observed in female offspring. Conversely, lower body fat percentages in female offspring have been shown in other studies [16, 19, 31]. Nonetheless, it is worth noting that body composition changes seem to be more prominent in male offspring. This is potentially because of a tendency for greater weight gain with aging; however, the exact reason for the sex-specific differences remains unknown [9].

With consideration of these inconsistencies, it is difficult to determine if offspring BW is a causal factor or is determined by alterations in the metabolic phenotype of the offspring. Interestingly, it has been observed that the alterations in BW, lean and fat mass are secondary to other metabolic improvements and often develop later in offspring life. For instance, improvements in glucose metabolism have been observed in multiple studies regardless of inconsistencies in BW and body composition changes between studies [16, 26, 29, 31]. This suggests that metabolic reprograming is, at least in part, independent of body composition changes and is more likely causal of these alterations with aging or subsequent metabolic challenges (i.e., overnutrition). Accordingly, significantly smaller BW and fat mass gains were observed in sedentary pups from exercised mothers who were fed a high-fat-high-sugar diet (HFHS) compared to HFHS-diet fed pups from non-exercising mothers [17, 20]. This suggests that subsequent nutritional manipulations in offspring may be needed to elicit changes in BW and body composition and to better understand the relationship between changes in BW and metabolic reprogramming.

### *2.2.2 Glucose tolerance*

Since SkM and liver metabolic alterations have a profound impact on the development of systemic metabolic disease, it is important to address how maternal exercise alters metabolism of these tissues. Exercise prior to and during pregnancy increases glucose tolerance and insulin sensitivity across offspring lifespan independent of changes in BW [16, 17, 19, 26, 27, 30, 31] and persist in second generation progeny [32]. Interestingly, in offspring from metabolically healthy exercising mothers, improvements in glucose tolerance are mostly observed in adulthood of the animal rather than early stages of life (i.e., at weaning) [16, 18, 25, 26]. This might be the case considering that the effects of maternal exercise are "diluted" in offspring from metabolically healthy mothers, and therefore these effects might be more pronounced in offspring from mothers with obesity, considering the previously described metabolic derangements that maternal obesity elicits. Accordingly, offspring and maternal glucose intolerance stemming from maternal obesity can be rescued by maternal pregestational and gestation exercise, and this effect is evident in early offspring life [18, 25, 29–31, 33]. These findings suggest that maternal exercise could enhance the ability of offspring to resist the future development of IR; however, these improvements may not be readily observed in healthy offspring before adulthood or without a subsequent metabolic challenge.

Multiple *in vivo* and *in vitro* techniques have been used in studies to confirm that enhanced glucose disposal stems from improved offspring peripheral (i.e., SkM) insulin sensitivity as a result of maternal exercise. Improved insulin sensitivity in offspring from obese mothers seems to be driven by an increase in SkM GLUT4 expression [16, 18, 23, 26, 27]; however, improved glucose tolerance independent of the changes in GLUT4 expression has similarly been observed [29, 31]. This indicates that an improvement in glucose transport capacity is not the only mechanism responsible for improved glucose clearance. Offspring from exercising compared to sedentary mothers exhibit improved SkM insulin signaling cascade activation with insulin stimulation; this is evidenced by higher phosphorylation of Protein Kinase B, also known as AKT, a key mediator of insulin-stimulated glucose uptake [17]. In addition to the effects of maternal exercise on SkM, it is important to recognize that these adaptations extend to offspring liver, a major organ for regulating glucose disposal and production. Maternal exercise improves mature offspring hepatic insulin sensitivity and lowers hepatic glucose production during hyperinsulinemic-euglycemic clamp [16]. Similar effects have been observed in an *in vitro* model where isolated hepatocytes of offspring from exercising mothers exhibit enhanced glucose control across basal and insulin- and glucagon-stimulated states [31]. Greater glucagon-mediated hepatocyte glucose production and insulin-mediated inhibition of glucose production suggest that maternal exercise improves liver glucose metabolism across different physiologic states (fasted vs. fed) [31]. Interestingly, it is worth noting that this effect is observed in offspring from exercising mothers independent of maternal metabolic status (healthy or obese). This suggests that while metabolic enhancements may be present, they may not be evident with measurements at the whole-organism level considering the multifaceted input of several organs [31]. In rodent models, it is clear, that maternal exercise negates the effects of maternal obesity through enhancements in offspring glucose metabolism, which lowers the potential for glycemic dysregulation in subsequent generations.

#### *2.2.3 Mitochondrial remodeling*

Maternal exercise lowers SkM and liver triglyceride content in offspring from both healthy and obese mothers [24, 29, 31]. Lower SkM and liver triglyceride content will decrease the chance of lipid accumulation-induced impairments with insulin signaling and are suggestive of an enhanced oxidative capacity. Maternal exercise increases offspring SkM mitochondrial density, length, and mitochondrial DNA content [19, 34]. These mitochondrial alterations predominantly stem from the effects of maternal exercise on PGC-1α, a key mediator of mitochondrial functioning and biogenesis [19, 34]. Maternal exercise before and during pregnancy attenuates high-fat diet (HFD) induced PGC-1α promoter hypermethylation in offspring SkM, and is able to rescue a HFD induced decrease in PGC-1α gene expression [19, 27]. Interestingly, the effect of maternal exercise on PGC-1α expression has only been observed in adult offspring [27]. This, however, may be an artifact of the rapid proliferation and differentiation of SkM cells during early growth compared to mature SkM, when myogenic cells are quiescent and transcription of genes is predominantly influenced by gene methylation [27]. Higher PGC-1α expression in SkM increases expression of its downstream targets including cytochrome C, a central component of the electron transport chain, which potentiates improvements in the regulation of oxidative phosphorylation [27]. Additionally, in SkM of offspring from exercising mothers, greater cytochrome C oxidase and citrate synthase activities have been observed [34], suggesting that maternal exercise has an effect on mitochondrial oxidative capacity. It is worth noting that similar hypermethylation and lower mRNA expression of PGC-1α is seen in SkM of individuals with T2D [35]. This points to maternal exercise as a potential therapy to ameliorate the transgenerational transmission of mitochondrial dysfunction in humans, by increasing the oxidative capacity as well.

In liver, the maternal exercise induced increase in PGC-1α mRNA expression is accompanied by higher protein expression of phosphorylated AMP-activated protein kinase (AMPK), which is considered to be a master regulator of energy metabolism [36]. This AMPK-PGC-1α axis and its increase is paralleled by an increase in PPARα mRNA expression and is suggestive of a greater potential for fatty acid oxidation.

Specifically, maternal exercise enhances gene expression of Acox1 and Acacb, enzymes involved in fatty acid handling and oxidation [36]. Interestingly, while improving the capacity for fatty acid oxidation, maternal exercise simultaneously decreases the potential for fatty acid storage by lowering PPARγ mRNA expression, a gene associated with hepatic steatosis [36, 37]. Further, greater phosphorylated AMPK expression in offspring from exercising mothers leads to greater phosphorylation of acetyl-CoA carboxylase which lowers the availability of malonyl-CoA, a precursor for fatty acid synthesis [36]. It is important to note that these adaptations on a cellular level extend to elicit whole-body protection and lead to lower BW gain and hepatic steatosis after pups are challenged with an obesogenic diet [36]. Overall, maternal exercise driven improvements of offspring mitochondrial bioenergetics are often seen as vital for proper metabolic functioning and resilience to metabolic challenges in adult life. These adaptations could influence the predisposition for the development of metabolic disease by altering mitochondrial substrate "preference" and oxidation capacity.

Maternal exercise increases the affinity for pyruvate and palmitoyl-CoA in offspring SkM mitochondria suggesting easier access of these substrates for the oxidative phosphorylation system (OXPHOS) [17]. Further, maternal exercise has no effect on the $K_m$ for palmitoyl-carnitine, which suggests that maternal exercise might be acting specifically on CPT-1, a commonly altered enzyme in obesity-related diseases. Finally, a larger decrease in enzyme affinity is seen for palmitoyl-CoA compared to pyruvate suggesting that maternal exercise increases offspring SkM preference for fatty acid oxidation and potentially explains the previously described decrease in triglyceride content [17, 29]. In addition to altering SkM metabolic pathways, offspring from exercising mothers exhibit greater levels of liver mRNA expression of genes involved in pyruvate metabolism (Pklr, Pcx), the tricarboxylic acid cycle (Pdha1, Pdk4, CS, Idh3a, Mdh2), and fatty acid transport and oxidation (Cd36, Fatp4, Acox, Cpt1) [31]. Together, this data shows that maternal exercise induces an array of adaptations that enhance substrate handling and subsequently increase resilience against future metabolic disease.

Data regarding maternal exercise and offspring OXPHOS capacity is limited. Maternal exercise decreases complex II and III activity and increases complex IV activity [22]. Additionally, when ADP-stimulated respiration is measured in SkM mitochondria from offspring of exercising mothers, there seems to be no effect on complex I and complex I + II respiration; however, data regarding respiration through complex II only is inconsistent with maternal exercise resulting in a decrease or having no effect on complex II maximal respiration [22, 23]. Interestingly, in isolated liver mitochondria from offspring of exercising mothers, lower complex II and higher complex IV activity and content is observed, and accompanied by lower maximal respiration through complex I, II, and I + II. Interestingly, respiratory control ratio (RCR) is lower in offspring mitochondria from both liver and SkM when respiration is supported through complex I and complex I + II [22]. As an index of how coupled respiration is to ADP phosphorylation, this would suggest a lower capacity for phosphorylating respiration to offset electron leak; however, implications about the effect of maternal exercise on offspring mitochondrial efficiency cannot be made as RCR, when used as a proxy of mitochondrial coupling, does not always match the ATP/O ratio, which is a direct measure of mitochondrial coupling [38]. Data regarding alterations in offspring energy efficiency come from oxygen consumption rates in free living conditions. Accordingly, on the level of the whole organism, maternal exercise increases the basal oxygen consumption rate, subsequently protecting offspring from overnutrition-induced obesity by increasing their energy expenditure [20, 30] Together, the limited data suggests that maternal exercise results in adaptations in mitochondrial respiration, but no conclusive remarks can be made considering the inconsistencies between and limited number of studies.

#### *2.2.4 Mitochondrial redox balance*

While mitochondria are often described predominantly in the light of energy metabolism, it is important to recognize their function in maintaining redox homeostasis. Mitochondria are mediators of redox balance, and this is influenced by alterations to pro- and antioxidant systems. Disruption of the redox balance due to alterations in mitochondrial bioenergetics or the redox buffering capacity are considered to be an integral part in the etiology of metabolic disease (i.e., IR) [39]. Maternal exercise lowers hydrogen peroxide production with complex II only and complex I + II supporting substrates in both SkM and liver mitochondria [22]; however, the effects seen in SkM are inconsistent across studies indicating maternal exercise may not affect hydrogen peroxide emission [23]. Interestingly, SkM and liver mitochondria from offspring of exercising mothers are protected from reverse electron transport linked hydrogen peroxide emission [22]. Hydrogen peroxide emission via reverse electron flow is often associated with overnutrition and suggests that maternal exercise has a protective effect on offspring redox balance during future metabolic challenges such as overnutrition [39]. In addition to lower hydrogen peroxide emission and subsequently lower reactive oxygen species (ROS) production, maternal exercise enhances glutathione activity in blood and liver [22]. Further, offspring from exercising mothers have lower blood thiol content suggestive of a higher antioxidant capacity. These adaptations are paralleled with higher offspring liver alpha-tocopherol which increases free radical scavenging ability and decreases lipid peroxidation [40–42]. Maternal exercise further induces a mitochondrial fatty acid profile shift by increasing short-chain and decreasing long-chain fatty acid content [22]. These changes can be beneficial considering that short-chain fatty acids are more resistant to free radical attack and peroxidation and have a positive influence on redox signaling [43, 44]. Finally, maternal exercises increases offspring LON protease (an oxidative stress induced mitochondrial degradation catalyst) and TFAM induced autophagy; these changes are suggestive of a greater mitochondrial turnover rate and overall lower susceptibility to oxidative stress induced mitochondrial dysfunction [24, 34]. Together, these findings suggest that maternal exercise increases antioxidant capacity, decreases ROS production, and lowers the potential accumulation of less functional mitochondria in offspring.

Together, maternal exercise will protect offspring from maternal obesity induced metabolic derangements and has the capacity to increase offspring resilience against future metabolic challenges. Further, offspring metabolic adaptations (**Figure 1**) as a result of maternal exercise seem to be independent of body composition alterations. These adaptations include improvements in offspring glucose and fatty acid metabolism across two major metabolically active tissues, the liver and SkM. In part, these adaptations are linked to mitochondrial structure remodeling, enhanced bioenergetic function, and greater redox capacity. Finally, it is imperative to keep in mind that cellular metabolic programing precedes improvements detected at the whole-body level making *in vitro* assessments indispensable for the understanding of maternal exercise-induced fetal programing.

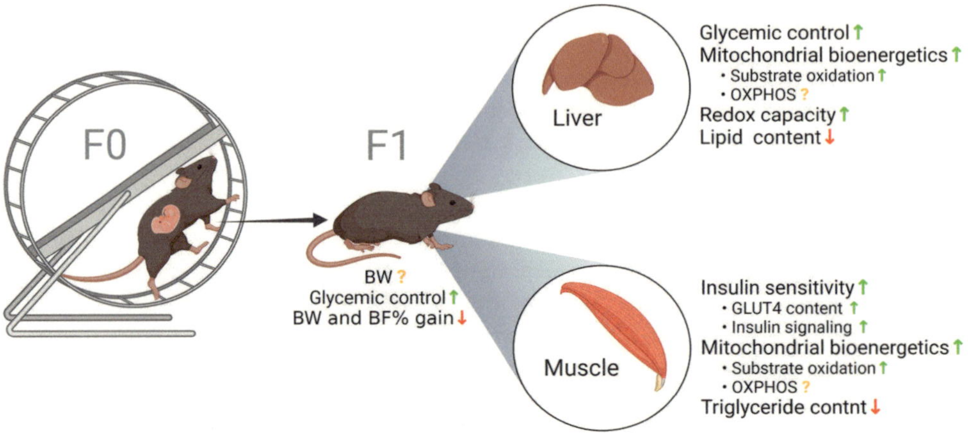


**Figure 1.**
*Maternal exercise enhances offspring metabolism across two major metabolically active tissues, the liver and SkM. Offspring from exercising mothers have lower body weight (BW) and body fat (BF%) gain with age and exhibit enhanced whole body glucose tolerance. Additionally, maternal exercise leads to greater insulin sensitivity, mitochondrial remodeling, and improved bioenergetic function and substrate metabolism in peripheral tissue. Abbreviations: BW, body weight; BF%, body fat percentage; and OXPHOS, oxidative phosphorylation.*

## 3. Human studies of maternal obesity and exercise effects on offspring metabolism

### 3.1 Effects of maternal obesity on offspring metabolism

While rodent models provide an insight into the effects of maternal exercise on progeny, a major obstacle is analogizing human and animal research considering the vast physiological difference between species. In humans, maternal obesity rates are rising and are in parallel with those of the general population [45, 46]. Pre-pregnancy obesity is likely to translate into excessive gestational weight gain, pre-eclampsia, gestational diabetes, and a greater propensity towards postpartum weight retention [47]. Moreover, maternal obesity increases the risk for congenital anomalies, fetal death, stillbirth, and neonatal, perinatal, and infant death [48, 49]. Increased maternal pre-pregnancy body mass index corelates with increased risk of offspring obesity [50]. Specifically, maternal obesity increases the odds of offspring obesity by 264%, while maternal overweight increases odds by 89% [50]. Neonates born to obese mothers are often large for gestational age with increased adiposity being a major determinant of fetal overgrowth [47]. Besides increasing adiposity, neonates of obese mothers have a higher propensity towards IR independent of maternal glycemia [51, 52]. Finally, maternal obesity is associated with an adverse lipid profile in offspring and an inclination towards the development of metabolic syndrome [53–55]. While this relationship between maternal and offspring metabolism is readily accepted, limitations in the understanding of epigenetic mechanisms governing infant metabolic reprograming remain. Moreover, the biological mechanisms behind metabolic adaptations that govern offspring metabolic phenotypes remain to be elucidated.

The use of umbilical cord derived mesenchymal stem cells (MSCs) has been recognized as a model for the investigation of metabolic programming of the human offspring donor. This model capitalizes on the multilineage potential of MSCs and their ability to differentiate into various lineages of mesenchymal tissue (muscle, fat, etc.) [56–61]. The phenotype of MSCs reflects that of the donor rendering it as an advantageous *in vitro* model to study offspring phenotypes on a molecular level [62–66]. MSCs from offspring of obese mothers exhibit a greater potential for adipogenesis associated with greater PPAR-γ, FABP4, and lipid content in adipogenically differentiated cells [65]. Further, evidence of lower β-catenin protein content paired with a lower inhibitory phosphorylation of GSK-3β in undifferentiated MSCs suggests a greater shift in cell commitment towards an adipocyte rather than myocyte lineage and will subsequently increase the propensity of the fetus towards greater adiposity [65]. Accordingly, greater MSC adipogenesis potential is positively correlated with infant body fat mass [65]. In line with greater potential for fetal adiposity, MSCs from offspring of obese mothers exhibit greater lipid accumulation and lower capacity for fatty acid oxidation when undergoing myogenesis, which will potentiate ectopic lipid accretion [64]. It is worth noting that fatty acid oxidation in MSCs from offspring of obese mothers is "less efficient" with more substrate flux towards incomplete rather than complete oxidation [64, 66]. Additionally, maternal obesity induces a MSC phenotype with lower metabolic flexibility and a decreased ability to meet metabolic demands, demonstrating primary deficits in fatty acid oxidation [66]. These factors have previously been observed in SkM of humans with non-gravid obesity and have been associated with the development of IR [67–69]. This suggests that maternal obesity may alter offspring metabolism with a predisposition towards metabolic disease (i.e., obesity). Accordingly, beta-oxidation decrements in myogenically differentiated MSCs from offspring of obese mothers are correlated with infant adiposity suggesting that fetal adiposity is in part predetermined by alterations in the fetal metabolic phenotype [63]. These inherent differences in MSC lipid metabolism seemingly stem from differential mitochondrial expression and methylation of genes involved in mitochondrial fatty acid metabolism and respiration (i.e., OXPHOS) and are correlated with neonatal adiposity [62, 63]. Particularly, alterations in lipid metabolism are associated with lower AMPK content and activation and hypermethylation of genes involved in fatty acid oxidation (i.e., ACC2, CPT1A) [64]. Overall, this data suggests that maternal obesity reprograms the offspring metabolic phenotype by increasing propensity towards adiposity, which, in part, occurs through the lowering of oxidative capacity. Moreover, considering that similar alterations are seen with non-gravid obesity, it is reasonable to postulate that this phenotype will predispose offspring to metabolic perturbations later in life. Accordingly, it is necessary to further our understanding of lifestyle interventions that could counteract the intergenerational transmission of metabolic disease. Specifically, non-pharmacological interventions, such as exercise could have a tremendous impact on fetal metabolic programing with overall metabolic disease lowering properties highlighting the need for more research studies. While alterations of the MSC phenotype as a consequence of maternal obesity have been shown, the effects of maternal exercise on offspring metabolic reprogramming remain understudied in humans, especially on a molecular level.

### 3.2 Effects of gestational exercise on offspring metabolism

Prenatal maternal exercise elicits an array of positive benefits for both mother and offspring. Maternal aerobic exercise lowers the risk for the development of gestational diabetes mellitus and lowers gestational weight gain in both healthy and mothers with gestational diabetes [5, 7, 8, 70]. Further, there is an inverse relationship between gestational weight gain and exercise duration and volume with benefits increasing as exercise volume approaches American College of Obstetricians and Gynecologists

(ACOG) recommendations of 500 MET-minute weekly [7, 8, 71]. Maternal exercise alone reduces the risk of macrosomia and offspring being large for gestational age without increasing risk of pre-term birth or low birth weight [8, 72, 73]. Further, maternal exercise may have a greater influence on birth weight reduction in maternal obesity, however, evidence remains weak [72, 73]. Similarly, the association of maternal exercise and birth weight remains weeak across multiple meta-analysis including women of all body mass index categories and seems to be driven predominantly by exercise volume [8, 72, 73]. Accordingly, the exercise-induced reduction of offspring birth weight is predominantly observed with exercise volumes over 810 MET-min, which is much greater than the 500 MET-min per week recommendation by ACOG [72]. Finally, birth weight reductions observed with maternal exercise are often not clinically significant (i.e., >300 g) making it hard to conclude if prenatal exercise has a significant effect on fetal birth weight [74, 75]. Additionally, while body weight can be influenced by fat and lean mass, maternal exercise does not seem to effect child morphometrics based on two recent meta-analyses [73, 76]. Nonetheless, while alterations in birth weight are not significant, there is evidence to support the beneficial effects of a prenatal healthy lifestyle (i.e., normal BMI, regular exercise, etc.) on the risk of offspring childhood (child age of 9–14) obesity [77]. Overall, while prenatal exercise influences maternal gestational weight gain, the effects of maternal exercise on offspring birth weight and body composition seem to be minimal. Accordingly, and in line with rodent studies, exercise induced body composition alterations might be secondary to other metabolic improvements and may decrease the risk of obesity development with aging.

The positive effects of exercise extend to maternal metabolic health through improvements in lipid and glucose metabolism. Data suggests that maternal exercise improves maternal metabolism during pregnancy and subsequently alters pregnancy outcomes and the metabolic phenotype of offspring. Physical activity during pregnancy reduces the rise of low density lipoprotein and triglyceride, and lowers delivery and neonatal complications [78–82]. Maternal blood lipids are associated with infant adiposity and alterations in MSC metabolism in offspring from mothers with obesity [63, 64, 78] suggesting a potential *in-utero* influence of maternal lipids on fetal metabolic programing. Recently shown, maternal aerobic exercise during gestation may alter the MSC phenotype, however, improvements in lipid oxidation, oxidation efficiency or uptake, and accumulation were not significant [83]. While the lack of effect is surprising based on previously described effects in rodent models and MSCs from offspring of mothers with obesity, it must be noted that exercising mothers were seemingly healthy and thus potentially "diluting" the effect of maternal exercise on offspring metabolic reprograming. Accordingly, the positive effects of maternal exercise on offspring MSC lipid metabolism may be pronounced in situations where an adverse intrauterine environment is instilled by maternal metabolic disease (i.e., obesity) [63–65, 83]; however, there are currently no studies exploring these effects.

Aerobic exercise during pregnancy significantly improves maternal glucose metabolism with a greater effect in women with overweight, obesity, and gestational diabetes [84, 85]. In particular, maternal aerobic exercise lowers insulin levels late in pregnancy and reduces the increase in blood insulin levels from 15- to 36-weeks of gestation [86]. Maternal dysglycemia, with or without gestational or type 2 diabetes, has been associated with adverse pregnancy outcomes (i.e., preeclampsia), offspring outcomes (i.e., excessive fetal growth, congenital abnormalities), and an overall increase in postpartum risk of development of T2D in both mother and offspring [87–89]. Evidence for maternal dysglycemia altering offspring metabolism can be further observed at the level of MSCs where metabolic derangements coincide with derangements in maternal glycemic control (i.e., HOMA-IR) [64]. Further, maternal aerobic exercise increases insulin-mediated glycogen synthesis rates in undifferentiated MSCs suggestive of greater insulin sensitivity [83]. This effect was paralleled with greater insulin-mediated phosphorylation of signaling marker GSK-3β in undifferentiated MSCs. Together, these promising effects could counter the previously described transmission of IR in the case of maternal glucose dysglycemia (i.e., during obesity). In addition to glycogen synthesis, enhanced glucose oxidation efficiency and partitioning of glucose towards oxidation is observed in both undifferentiated and myogenically differentiated MSCs from offspring of aerobically trained mothers. Interestingly, a trend towards a greater capacity for glucose oxidation was observed in myogenically differentiated but not undifferentiated MSCs [83]. It is worth noting that there is greater expression of complex I in myogenically differentiated MSCs, which could in part influence the greater glucose oxidation rates considering that glucose oxidation increases the input of electrons to complex I of mitochondria [83]; however, this effect needs to be further elucidated. As previously described, obesity driven metabolic derangements lead to less efficient mitochondria with a lower oxidative capacity; thus, it is possible that a greater capacity to oxidize glucose may attenuate the transmission of decrements in glucose metabolism across generations. The partitioning of glucose towards oxidation, rather than glycolytic intermediates (i.e., lactate), would lower the propensity towards metabolic disease considering that a lower oxidation capacity and greater lactate production have been linked with T2D [90–92]. While this data is associative in nature, the importance of exercise in improving the metabolism of both mother and offspring is clear (**Figure 2**).

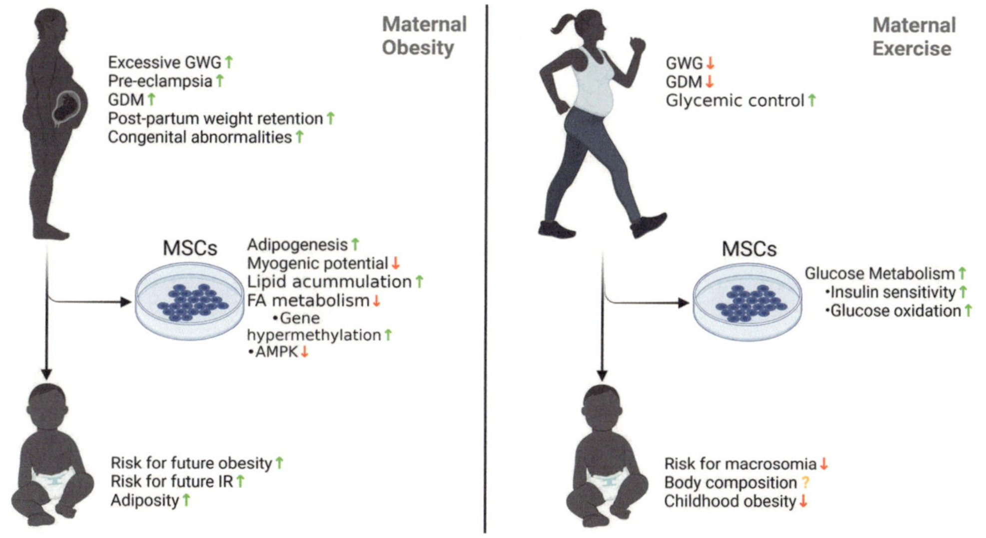


**Figure 2.**
*Maternal obesity increases pregnancy complications and introduces an array of metabolic derangements in mother and offspring health. Maternal gestational exercise improves many aspects of obesity-induced metabolic alterations and enhances maternal and offspring metabolism. Abbreviations: GWG, gestational weight gain; GDM, gestational diabetes mellitus; MSCs, mesenchymal stem cells; FA, fatty acid; AMPK, AMP-activated protein kinase; and IR, insulin resistance.*

## 4. Transfer of maternal exercise induced effects on offspring and exercise modalities

The effects of exercise, both acute and chronic, are partly mediated through the production and secretion of bioactive molecules termed cytokines. With exercise, an array of these metabolic factors are released by SkM influencing muscle metabolism as well as crosstalk between SkM and other organs. While extensive reviews have been published on this topic [93, 94], it is worth mentioning that these factors could mediate fetal programing as well. However, this is contingent on their placental blood barrier permeability. Many cytokines (i.e., IL-15, BAIBA, BDNF, Irisin, etc.) have an influence on energy metabolism and an overall positive effect on metabolic disease [93, 94]; however, the involvement of these cytokines in regulating offspring metabolic phenotypes is not yet understood. Recently, the effects of cytokine apelin have been shown to drive maternal exercise-induced metabolic reprogramming in offspring [19, 95]. Maternal exercise elevates apelin signaling which facilitates fetal muscle development and subsequently increases PGC-1α promoter demethylation, mitochondrial biogenesis and remodeling, and mitochondrial capacity [95]. This data suggests that maternal exercise-induced cytokine release could have a direct effect on fetal development by inducing specific adaptations that will later shape offspring metabolism. Accordingly, it is reasonable to postulate that different modes of exercise, based on their differences in cytokine expression profiles and differential metabolic demands [96–98], could have differing effects on offspring metabolic reprograming.

Exercise modes separate into aerobic and muscular strength training where activity is performed against a low resistance for a longer time or against high resistance for a short duration, respectively. These exercise modalities differ in the adaptations they elicit and are driven by the different energetic demands experienced during activity. During an acute bout of exercise, substrate oxidation is predominantly driven by the intensity and duration of exercise. There is a shift from predominantly fatty acid oxidation during prolonged low-moderate intensity exercise towards an almost exclusive reliance on glycolytic substrates during high-intensity exercise bouts. Aerobic training is often associated with improvements in cardiorespiratory fitness via an increase in maximal oxygen consumption and mitochondrial biogenesis. Specifically, aerobic exercise increases SkM mitochondrial protein synthesis, density, and oxidative function, which subsequently improves endurance capacity [99]. With this, it is not surprising that aerobic exercise results in a greater abundance of proteins involved in mitochondrial ATP production, TCA cycle, transport, and oxidation of fatty acids which are predominantly regulated through PGC-1α expression [99]. In contrast, while the effects of resistance exercise on these parameters are minimal, resistance training increases muscle size, strength, myofibrillar protein synthesis, and anaerobic capacity significantly more than aerobic exercise [99]. Both modalities improve glucose handling and are beneficial for improving glucose control predominantly through enhancing insulin sensitivity (i.e., greater GLUT4 expression) [99–101]. Additionally, aerobic training improves cardiovascular profiles and decreases adiposity, while resistance training seemingly has a very limited effect on either of these parameters [99]. Overall, while both modalities reduce the risk and lower the derangements of metabolic disease (i.e., obesity), the effects by which aerobic and resistance training influence metabolism vary to a great extent. With this in mind, it is reasonable to postulate that depending on the maternal exercise mode, effects on offspring metabolic reprograming will differ; however, research directly comparing the effects of maternal exercise modes on offspring metabolic health outcomes remains scarce especially with maternal muscular strength training.

While muscular strength training during pregnancy is safe and recommended, most research assessing the effects of prenatal exercise on offspring metabolic health utilizes aerobic only or a combination of aerobic and strength training. While these two exercise modes are beneficial for both maternal and offspring health, a delineation of their independent effects on offspring metabolic health is currently not possible [70]. Further, a comparison of the independent effects of maternal aerobic or strength training on offspring metabolism is primarily limited due to the lack of the studies utilizing maternal strength training [69]. To date, it is shown that a combination of aerobic and strength training during pregnancy increases cardiorespiratory fitness and muscle strength more so than aerobic or strength training alone [70]. Further, combined training has the most significant impact on decreasing gestational weight gain; however, more studies are needed to confirm these findings [70]. Evidence is similarly weak with inconsistent findings on the effects of combined training on improvements in birth weight; however, it is important to note that all exercise interventions increase the chance of the offspring having a normal birth weight and reduce the risk of macrosomia [70]. In conclusion, gestational exercise is safe and recommended considering the resulting array of positive metabolic changes in both mother and offspring.

## 5. Conclusion

Considering the prevalence and burden of obesity and T2D in today's society, it is crucial to identify new targets and treatment approaches to combat these diseases. As discussed, maternal exercise before and/or during pregnancy has a critical influence on offspring metabolism and can decrease their risk of development of metabolic disease later in life. While the current understanding of the precise mechanisms underlying these developmental influences is not fully understood, future work in this area holds immense potential to prevent and alleviate instances of obesity and improve the life-long health of the child.

## Author details

Filip Jevtovic[1,2] and Linda May[1,2*]

1 Human Performance Laboratory, Department of Kinesiology, East Carolina University, Greenville, NC, United States

2 East Carolina Diabetes and Obesity Institute, East Carolina University, Greenville, NC, United States

*Address all correspondence to: mayl@ecu.edu

## References

[1] Pulgaron ER, Delamater AM. Obesity and type 2 diabetes in children: Epidemiology and treatment. Current Diabetes Reports. 2014;**14**:508. DOI: 10.1007/s11892-014-0508-y

[2] Sales VM, Ferguson-Smith AC, Patti M-E. Epigenetic mechanisms of transmission of metabolic disease across generations. Cell Metabolism. 2017;**25**:559-571. DOI: 10.1016/j.cmet.2017.02.016

[3] Beetham KS, Giles C, Noetel M, Clifton V, Jones JC, Naughton G. The effects of vigorous intensity exercise in the third trimester of pregnancy: A systematic review and meta-analysis. BMC Pregnancy and Childbirth. 2019;**19**:281. DOI: 10.1186/s12884-019-2441-1

[4] Davenport MH, Ruchat S-M, Poitras VJ, Jaramillo Garcia A, Gray CE, Barrowman N, et al. Prenatal exercise for the prevention of gestational diabetes mellitus and hypertensive disorders of pregnancy: A systematic review and meta-analysis. British Journal of Sports Medicine. 2018;**52**:1367-1375. DOI: 10.1136/bjsports-2018-099355

[5] Ming W-K, Ding W, Zhang CJP, Zhong L, Long Y, Li Z, et al. The effect of exercise during pregnancy on gestational diabetes mellitus in normal-weight women: A systematic review and meta-analysis. BMC Pregnancy and Childbirth. 2018;**18**:440. DOI: 10.1186/s12884-018-2068-7

[6] Moyer C, Reoyo OR, May L. The influence of prenatal exercise on offspring health: A review. Clinical Medicine Insights: Women's Health. 2016;**9**:CMWH.S34670. DOI: 10.4137/CMWH.S34670

[7] Wang J, Wen D, Liu X, Liu Y. Impact of exercise on maternal gestational weight gain: An updated meta-analysis of randomized controlled trials. Medicine. 2019;**98**:e16199. DOI: 10.1097/MD.0000000000016199

[8] Wiebe HW, Boulé NG, Chari R, Davenport MH. The effect of supervised prenatal exercise on fetal growth: A meta-analysis. Obstetrics & Gynecology. 2015;**125**:1185-1194. DOI: 10.1097/AOG.0000000000000801

[9] Kusuyama J, Alves-Wagner AB, Makarewicz NS, Goodyear LJ. Effects of maternal and paternal exercise on offspring metabolism. Nature Metabolism. 2020;**2**:858-872. DOI: 10.1038/s42255-020-00274-7

[10] Gniuli D, Calcagno A, Caristo ME, Mancuso A, Macchi V, Mingrone G, et al. Effects of high-fat diet exposure during fetal life on type 2 diabetes development in the progeny. Journal of Lipid Research. 2008;**49**:1936-1945. DOI: 10.1194/jlr.M800033-JLR200

[11] Masuyama H, Hiramatsu Y. Effects of a high-fat diet exposure in utero on the metabolic syndrome-like phenomenon in mouse offspring through epigenetic changes in adipocytokine gene expression. Endocrinology. 2012;**153**:2823-2830. DOI: 10.1210/en.2011-2161

[12] Samuelsson A-M, Matthews PA, Argenton M, Christie MR, McConnell JM, Jansen EHJM, et al. Diet-induced obesity in female mice leads to offspring hyperphagia, adiposity, hypertension, and insulin resistance: A novel murine model of developmental programming. Hypertension. 2008;**51**:383-392. DOI: 10.1161/HYPERTENSIONAHA.107.101477

[13] Bayol SA, Simbi BH, Stickland NC. A maternal cafeteria diet during gestation and lactation promotes adiposity and impairs skeletal muscle development and metabolism in rat offspring at weaning: Cafeteria diet in developing rats. The Journal of Physiology. 2005;**567**:951-961. DOI: 10.1113/jphysiol.2005.088989

[14] Latouche C, Heywood SE, Henry SL, Ziemann M, Lazarus R, El-Osta A, et al. Maternal overnutrition programs changes in the expression of skeletal muscle genes that are associated with insulin resistance and defects of oxidative phosphorylation in adult male rat offspring. The Journal of Nutrition. 2014;**144**:237-244. DOI: 10.3945/jn.113.186775

[15] Stenkula KG, Erlanson-Albertsson C. Adipose cell size: Importance in health and disease. American Journal of Physiology-Regulatory, Integrative and Comparative Physiology. 2018;**315**:R284-R295. DOI: 10.1152/ajpregu.00257.2017

[16] Carter LG, Qi NR, Cabo RD, Pearson KJ. Maternal exercise improves insulin sensitivity in mature rat offspring. Medicine & Science in Sports & Exercise. 2013;**45**:832-840. DOI: 10.1249/MSS.0b013e31827de953

[17] Quiclet C, Dubouchaud H, Berthon P, Sanchez H, Vial G, Siti F, et al. Maternal exercise modifies body composition and energy substrates handling in male offspring fed a high-fat/high-sucrose diet: Maternal exercise and offspring metabolism. The Journal of Physiology. 2017;**595**:7049-7062. DOI: 10.1113/JP274739

[18] Raipuria M, Bahari H, Morris MJ. Effects of maternal diet and exercise during pregnancy on glucose metabolism in skeletal muscle and fat of weanling rats. PLoS One. 2015;**10**:e0120980. DOI: 10.1371/journal.pone.0120980

[19] Son JS, Zhao L, Chen Y, Chen K, Chae SA, de Avila JM, et al. Maternal exercise via exerkine apelin enhances brown adipogenesis and prevents metabolic dysfunction in offspring mice. Science Advances. 2020;**6**:eaaz0359. DOI: 10.1126/sciadv.aaz0359

[20] Wasinski F, Bacurau RFP, Estrela GR, Klempin F, Arakaki AM, Batista RO, et al. Exercise during pregnancy protects adult mouse offspring from diet-induced obesity. Nutrition & Metabolism (London). 2015;**12**:56. DOI: 10.1186/s12986-015-0052-z

[21] Eclarinal JD, Zhu S, Baker MS, Piyarathna DB, Coarfa C, Fiorotto ML, et al. Maternal exercise during pregnancy promotes physical activity in adult offspring. The FASEB Journal. 2016;**30**:2541-2548. DOI: 10.1096/fj.201500018R

[22] Siti F, Dubouchaud H, Hininger I, Quiclet C, Vial G, Galinier A, et al. Maternal exercise before and during gestation modifies liver and muscle mitochondria in rat offspring. Journal of Experimental Biology. 2019;**222**:jeb.194969. DOI: 10.1242/jeb.194969

[23] Falcão-Tebas F, Marin EC, Kuang J, Bishop DJ, McConell GK. Maternal exercise attenuates the lower skeletal muscle glucose uptake and insulin secretion caused by paternal obesity in female adult rat offspring. The Journal of Physiology. 2020;**598**:4251-4270. DOI: 10.1113/JP279582

[24] Sheldon RD, Nicole Blaize A, Fletcher JA, Pearson KJ, Donkin SS, Newcomer SC, et al. Gestational exercise protects adult male offspring from high-fat diet-induced hepatic steatosis.

Journal of Hepatology. 2016;**64**:171-178. DOI: 10.1016/j.jhep.2015.08.022

[25] Vega CC, Reyes-Castro LA, Bautista CJ, Larrea F, Nathanielsz PW, Zambrano E. Exercise in obese female rats has beneficial effects on maternal and male and female offspring metabolism. International Journal of Obesity. 2015;**39**:712-719. DOI: 10.1038/ijo.2013.150

[26] Carter LG, Lewis KN, Wilkerson DC, Tobia CM, Ngo Tenlep SY, Shridas P, et al. Perinatal exercise improves glucose homeostasis in adult offspring. American Journal of Physiology-Endocrinology and Metabolism. 2012;**303**:E1061-E1068. DOI: 10.1152/ajpendo.00213.2012

[27] Laker RC, Lillard TS, Okutsu M, Zhang M, Hoehn KL, Connelly JJ, et al. Exercise prevents maternal high-fat diet–induced hypermethylation of the Pgc-1α gene and age-dependent metabolic dysfunction in the offspring. Diabetes. 2014;**63**:1605-1611. DOI: 10.2337/db13-1614

[28] Quiclet C, Siti F, Dubouchaud H, Vial G, Berthon P, Fontaine E, et al. Short-term and long-term effects of submaximal maternal exercise on offspring glucose homeostasis and pancreatic function. American Journal of Physiology-Endocrinology and Metabolism. 2016;**311**:E508-E518. DOI: 10.1152/ajpendo.00126.2016

[29] Stanford KI, Lee M-Y, Getchell KM, So K, Hirshman MF, Goodyear LJ. Exercise before and during pregnancy prevents the deleterious effects of maternal high-fat feeding on metabolic health of male offspring. Diabetes. 2015;**64**:427-433. DOI: 10.2337/db13-1848

[30] Zheng J, Alves-Wagner AB, Stanford KI, Prince NB, So K, Mul JD, et al. Maternal and paternal exercise regulate offspring metabolic health and beta cell phenotype. BMJ Open Diabetes Research & Care. 2020;**8**:e000890. DOI: 10.1136/bmjdrc-2019-000890

[31] Stanford KI, Takahashi H, So K, Alves-Wagner AB, Prince NB, Lehnig AC, et al. Maternal exercise improves glucose tolerance in female offspring. Diabetes. 2017;**66**:2124-2136. DOI: 10.2337/db17-0098

[32] Alves-Wagner AB, Kusuyama J, Nigro P, Ramachandran K, Makarewicz N, Hirshman MF, et al. Grandmaternal exercise improves metabolic health of second-generation offspring. Molecular Metabolism. 2022;**60**:101490. DOI: 10.1016/j.molmet.2022.101490

[33] Fernandez-Twinn DS, Gascoin G, Musial B, Carr S, Duque-Guimaraes D, Blackmore HL, et al. Exercise rescues obese mothers' insulin sensitivity, placental hypoxia and male offspring insulin sensitivity. Scientific Reports. 2017;7:44650. DOI: 10.1038/srep44650

[34] Liu J, Lee I, Feng H-Z, Galen SS, Hüttemann PP, Perkins GA, et al. Aerobic exercise preconception and during pregnancy enhances oxidative capacity in the hindlimb muscles of mice offspring. Journal of Strength and Conditioning Research. 2018;**32**:1391-1403. DOI: 10.1519/JSC.0000000000002416

[35] Barrès R, Osler ME, Yan J, Rune A, Fritz T, Caidahl K, et al. Non-CpG methylation of the PGC-1α promoter through DNMT3B controls mitochondrial density. Cell Metabolism. 2009;**10**:189-198. DOI: 10.1016/j.cmet.2009.07.011

[36] Kasper P, Breuer S, Hoffmann T, Vohlen C, Janoschek R, Schmitz L, et al. Maternal exercise mediates hepatic

metabolic programming via activation of AMPK-PGC1α axis in the offspring of obese mothers. Cell. 2021;**10**:1247. DOI: 10.3390/cells10051247

[37] Wang Y, Nakajima T, Gonzalez FJ, Tanaka N. PPARs as metabolic regulators in the liver: Lessons from liver-specific PPAR-null mice. IJMS. 2020;**21**:2061. DOI: 10.3390/ijms21062061

[38] Salin K, Villasevil EM, Anderson GJ, Selman C, Chinopoulos C, Metcalfe NB. The RCR and ATP/O indices can give contradictory messages about mitochondrial efficiency. Integrative and Comparative Biology. 2018;**58**:486-494. DOI: 10.1093/icb/icy085

[39] Fisher-Wellman KH, Neufer PD. Linking mitochondrial bioenergetics to insulin resistance via redox biology. Trends in Endocrinology and Metabolism. 2012;**23**:142-153. DOI: 10.1016/j.tem.2011.12.008

[40] Gavazza MB, Catalá A. The effect of α-tocopherol on lipid peroxidation of microsomes and mitochondria from rat testis. Prostaglandins, Leukotrienes and Essential Fatty Acids. 2006;**74**:247-254. DOI: 10.1016/j.plefa.2006.01.007

[41] Kogure K. Mechanism of potent antiperoxidative effect of capsaicin. Biochimica et Biophysica Acta (BBA). General Subjects. 2002;**1573**:84-92. DOI: 10.1016/S0304-4165(02)00335-5

[42] Şekeroğlu V, Aydın B, Atlı Şekeroğlu Z, Özdener KY. Hepatoprotective effects of capsaicin and alpha-tocopherol on mitochondrial function in mice fed a high-fat diet. Biomedicine & Pharmacotherapy. 2018;**98**:821-825. DOI: 10.1016/j.biopha.2018.01.026

[43] González-Bosch C, Boorman E, Zunszain PA, Mann GE. Short-chain fatty acids as modulators of redox signaling in health and disease. Redox Biology. 2021;**47**:102165. DOI: 10.1016/j.redox.2021.102165

[44] Hulbert AJ, Kelly MA, Abbott SK. Polyunsaturated fats, membrane lipids and animal longevity. Journal of Comparative Physiology. B. 2014;**184**:149-166. DOI: 10.1007/s00360-013-0786-8

[45] Driscoll AK, Gregory, Elizabeth CW. Increases in prepregnancy obesity: United States. 2020;**2016-2019**:8

[46] Heslehurst N, Ells L, Simpson H, Batterham A, Wilkinson J, Summerbell C. Trends in maternal obesity incidence rates, demographic predictors, and health inequalities in 36 821 women over a 15-year period. BJOG: An International Journal of Obstetrics & Gynaecology. 2007;**114**:187-194. DOI: 10.1111/j.1471-0528.2006.01180.x

[47] Catalano PM, Shankar K. Obesity and pregnancy: Mechanisms of short term and long term adverse consequences for mother and child. BMJ. 2017;**356**:j1. DOI: 10.1136/bmj.j1

[48] Aune D, Saugstad OD, Henriksen T, Tonstad S. Maternal body mass index and the risk of fetal death, stillbirth, and infant death: A systematic review and meta-analysis. JAMA. 2014;**311**:1536. DOI: 10.1001/jama.2014.2269

[49] Stothard KJ, Tennant PWG, Bell R, Rankin J. Maternal overweight and obesity and the risk of congenital anomalies: A systematic review and meta-analysis. Yearbook of Pediatrics. 2010;**2010**:451-453. DOI: 10.1016/S0084-3954(09)79344-3

[50] Heslehurst N, Vieira R, Akhter Z, Bailey H, Slack E, Ngongalah L, et al. The association between maternal body

mass index and child obesity: A systematic review and meta-analysis. PLoS Medicine. 2019;**16**:e1002817. DOI: 10.1371/journal.pmed.1002817

[51] Catalano PM, Presley L, Minium J, Hauguel-de MS. Fetuses of obese mothers develop insulin resistance in utero. Diabetes Care. 2009;**32**:1076-1080. DOI: 10.2337/dc08-2077

[52] HAPO Study Cooperative Research Group. Hyperglycaemia and Adverse Pregnancy Outcome (HAPO) Study: Associations with maternal body mass index: HAPO—BMI and perinatal outcomes. BJOG: An International Journal of Obstetrics & Gynaecology. 2010;**117**:575-584. DOI: 10.1111/j.1471-0528.2009.02486.x

[53] Boney CM, Verma A, Tucker R, Vohr BR. Metabolic syndrome in childhood: Association with birth weight, maternal obesity, and gestational diabetes mellitus. Pediatrics. 2005;**115**:e290-e296. DOI: 10.1542/peds.2004-1808

[54] Godfrey KM, Sheppard A, Gluckman PD, Lillycrop KA, Burdge GC, McLean C, et al. Epigenetic gene promoter methylation at birth is associated with child's later adiposity. Diabetes. 2011;**60**:1528-1534. DOI: 10.2337/db10-0979

[55] Hochner H, Friedlander Y, Calderon-Margalit R, Meiner V, Sagy Y, Avgil-Tsadok M, et al. Associations of maternal prepregnancy body mass index and gestational weight gain with adult offspring cardiometabolic risk factors: The jerusalem perinatal family follow-up study. Circulation. 2012;**125**:1381-1389. DOI: 10.1161/CIRCULATIONAHA.111.070060

[56] Gang EJ, Jeong JA, Hong SH, Hwang SH, Kim SW, Yang IH, et al. Skeletal myogenic differentiation of mesenchymal stem cells isolated from human umbilical cord blood. Stem Cells. 2004;**22**:617-624. DOI: 10.1634/stemcells.22-4-617

[57] Hong SH, Gang EJ, Jeong JA, Ahn C, Hwang SH, Yang IH, et al. In vitro differentiation of human umbilical cord blood-derived mesenchymal stem cells into hepatocyte-like cells. Biochemical and Biophysical Research Communications. 2005;**330**:1153-1161. DOI: 10.1016/j.bbrc.2005.03.086

[58] Pittenger MF, Mackay AM, Beck SC, Jaiswal RK, Douglas R, Mosca JD, et al. Multilineage potential of adult human mesenchymal stem cells. Science. 1999;**284**:143-147. DOI: 10.1126/science.284.5411.143

[59] Shapiro ALB, Boyle KE, Dabelea D, Patinkin ZW, De la Houssaye B, Ringham BM, et al. Nicotinamide promotes adipogenesis in umbilical cord-derived mesenchymal stem cells and is associated with neonatal adiposity: The healthy start BabyBUMP project. PLoS One. 2016;**11**:e0159575. DOI: 10.1371/journal.pone.0159575

[60] Witt R, Weigand A, Boos AM, Cai A, Dippold D, Boccaccini AR, et al. Mesenchymal stem cells and myoblast differentiation under HGF and IGF-1 stimulation for 3D skeletal muscle tissue engineering. BMC Cell Biology. 2017;**18**:15. DOI: 10.1186/s12860-017-0131-2

[61] Yu Y, Song Y, Chen Y, Zhang F, Qi F. Differentiation of umbilical cord mesenchymal stem cells into hepatocytes in comparison with bone marrow mesenchymal stem cells. Molecular Medicine Reports. 2018;**18**:2009-2016. DOI: 10.3892/mmr.2018.9181

[62] Baker PR, Patinkin ZW, Shapiro ALB, de la Houssaye BA,

Janssen RC, Vanderlinden LA, et al. Altered gene expression and metabolism in fetal umbilical cord mesenchymal stem cells correspond with differences in 5-month-old infant adiposity gain. Scientific Reports. 2017;7:18095. DOI: 10.1038/s41598-017-17588-4

[63] Baker PR, Patinkin Z, Shapiro ALB, De La Houssaye BA, Woontner M, Boyle KE, et al. Maternal obesity and increased neonatal adiposity correspond with altered infant mesenchymal stem cell metabolism. JCI Insight. 2017;**2**:e94200. DOI: 10.1172/jci.insight.94200

[64] Boyle KE, Patinkin ZW, Shapiro ALB, Bader C, Vanderlinden L, Kechris K, et al. Maternal obesity alters fatty acid oxidation, AMPK activity, and associated DNA methylation in mesenchymal stem cells from human infants. Molecular Metabolism. 2017;**6**:1503-1516. DOI: 10.1016/j.molmet.2017.08.012

[65] Boyle KE, Patinkin ZW, Shapiro ALB, Baker PR, Dabelea D, Friedman JE. Mesenchymal stem cells from infants born to obese mothers exhibit greater potential for adipogenesis: The healthy start BabyBUMP project. Diabetes. 2016;**65**:647-659. DOI: 10.2337/db15-0849

[66] Erickson ML, Patinkin ZW, Duensing AM, Dabelea D, Redman LM, Boyle KE. Maternal metabolic health drives mesenchymal stem cell metabolism and infant fat mass at birth. JCI Insight. 2021;**6**:e146606. DOI: 10.1172/jci.insight.146606

[67] Bell JA, Reed MA, Consitt LA, Martin OJ, Haynie KR, Hulver MW, et al. Lipid partitioning, incomplete fatty acid oxidation, and insulin signal transduction in primary human muscle cells: Effects of severe obesity, fatty acid incubation, and fatty acid translocase/CD36 overexpression. The Journal of Clinical Endocrinology & Metabolism. 2010;**95**:3400-3410. DOI: 10.1210/jc.2009-1596

[68] Houmard JA. Intramuscular lipid oxidation and obesity. American Journal of Physiology-Regulatory, Integrative and Comparative Physiology. 2008;**294**:R1111-R1116. DOI: 10.1152/ajpregu.00396.2007

[69] Koves TR, Ussher JR, Noland RC, Slentz D, Mosedale M, Ilkayeva O, et al. Mitochondrial overload and incomplete fatty acid oxidation contribute to skeletal muscle insulin resistance. Cell Metabolism. 2008;**7**:45-56. DOI: 10.1016/j.cmet.2007.10.013

[70] Perales M, Santos-Lozano A, Ruiz JR, Lucia A, Barakat R. Benefits of aerobic or resistance training during pregnancy on maternal health and perinatal outcomes: A systematic review. Early Human Development. 2016;**94**:43-48. DOI: 10.1016/j.earlhumdev.2016.01.004

[71] Committee on Obstetric Practice. Physical Activity and Exercise During Pregnancy and the Postpartum Period. 2020;**135**:11

[72] Chen Y, Ma G, Hu Y, Yang Q, Deavila JM, Zhu M-J, et al. Effects of maternal exercise during pregnancy on perinatal growth and childhood obesity outcomes: A meta-analysis and meta-regression. Sports Medicine. 2021;**51**:2329-2347. DOI: 10.1007/s40279-021-01499-6

[73] Davenport MH, Meah VL, Ruchat S-M, Davies GA, Skow RJ, Barrowman N, et al. Impact of prenatal exercise on neonatal and childhood outcomes: A systematic review and meta-analysis. British Journal of Sports Medicine. 2018;**52**:1386-1396. DOI: 10.1136/bjsports-2018-099836

[74] Bell R, Palma S. Antenatal exercise and birthweight. The Australian & New Zealand Journal of Obstetrics & Gynaecology. 2000;**40**:70-73. DOI: 10.1111/j.1479-828X.2000.tb03171.x

[75] Guillemette L, Hay JL, Kehler DS, Hamm NC, Oldfield C, McGavock JM, et al. Exercise in pregnancy and children's cardiometabolic risk factors: A systematic review and meta-analysis. Sports Medicine—Open. 2018;**4**:35. DOI: 10.1186/s40798-018-0148-x

[76] McPherson N, Lane M, Sandeman L, Owens J, Fullston T. An exercise-only intervention in obese fathers restores glucose and insulin regulation in conjunction with the rescue of pancreatic islet cell morphology and MicroRNA expression in male offspring. Nutrients. 2017;**9**:122. DOI: 10.3390/nu9020122

[77] Dhana K, Haines J, Liu G, Zhang C, Wang X, Field AE, et al. Association between maternal adherence to healthy lifestyle practices and risk of obesity in offspring: Results from two prospective cohort studies of mother-child pairs in the United States. BMJ. 2018;**362**:k2486. DOI: 10.1136/bmj.k2486

[78] Geraghty AA, Alberdi G, O'Sullivan EJ, O'Brien EC, Crosbie B, Twomey PJ, et al. Maternal blood lipid profile during pregnancy and associations with child adiposity: Findings from the ROLO study. PLoS One. 2016;**11**:e0161206. DOI: 10.1371/journal.pone.0161206

[79] Jin W-Y, Lin S-L, Hou R-L, Chen X-Y, Han T, Jin Y, et al. Associations between maternal lipid profile and pregnancy complications and perinatal outcomes: A population-based study from China. BMC Pregnancy and Childbirth. 2016;**16**:60. DOI: 10.1186/s12884-016-0852-9

[80] Ramírez-Vélez R, Lobelo F, Aguilar-de Plata AC, Izquierdo M, García-Hermoso A. Exercise during pregnancy on maternal lipids: A secondary analysis of randomized controlled trial. BMC Pregnancy and Childbirth. 2017;**17**:396. DOI: 10.1186/s12884-017-1571-6

[81] Strom CJ, McDonald SM, Remchak M-M, Kew KA, Rushing BR, Houmard JA, et al. The influence of maternal aerobic exercise, blood DHA and EPA concentrations on maternal lipid profiles. IJERPH. 2022;**19**:3550. DOI: 10.3390/ijerph19063550

[82] Zheng W, Zhang L, Tian Z, Zhang L, Liang X, Li G. Establishing reference ranges of serum lipid level during pregnancy and evaluating its association with perinatal outcomes: A cohort study. International Journal of Gynecology & Obstetrics. 2022;**156**:361-369. DOI: 10.1002/ijgo.13636

[83] Chaves AB, Weyrauch LA, Zheng D, Biagioni EM, Krassovskaia PM, Davidson BL, et al. Influence of maternal exercise on glucose and lipid metabolism in offspring stem cells: ENHANCED by Mom. The Journal of Clinical Endocrinology & Metabolism. 2022;**107**:dgac270. DOI: 10.1210/clinem/dgac270

[84] Davenport MH, Sobierajski F, Mottola MF, Skow RJ, Meah VL, Poitras VJ, et al. Glucose responses to acute and chronic exercise during pregnancy: A systematic review and meta-analysis. British Journal of Sports Medicine. 2018;**52**:1357-1366. DOI: 10.1136/bjsports-2018-099829

[85] McDonald SM, May LE, Hinkle SN, Grantz KL, Zhang C. Maternal moderate-to-vigorous physical activity before and during pregnancy and maternal glucose tolerance: Does timing matter? Medicine

& Science in Sports & Exercise. 2021. DOI: 10.1249/MSS.0000000000002730

[86] McDonald SM, Strom C, Remchak M, Chaves A, Broskey NT, Isler C, et al. The effects of aerobic exercise on markers of maternal metabolism during pregnancy. Birth Defects Research. 2021;**113**:227-237. DOI: 10.1002/bdr2.1780

[87] Farrar D, Simmonds M, Bryant M, Sheldon TA, Tuffnell D, Golder S, et al. Hyperglycaemia and risk of adverse perinatal outcomes: systematic review and meta-analysis. BMJ. 2016;**354**:i4694. DOI: 10.1136/bmj.i4694

[88] Silva CM, Arnegard ME, Maric-Bilkan C. Dysglycemia in pregnancy and maternal/fetal outcomes. Journal of Women's Health. 2021;**30**:187-193. DOI: 10.1089/jwh.2020.8853

[89] Yamamoto JM, Kellett JE, Balsells M, García-Patterson A, Hadar E, Solà I, et al. Gestational diabetes mellitus and diet: A systematic review and meta-analysis of randomized controlled trials examining the impact of modified dietary interventions on maternal glucose control and neonatal birth weight. Diabetes Care. 2018;**41**:1346-1361. DOI: 10.2337/dc18-0102

[90] Jones TE, Pories WJ, Houmard JA, Tanner CJ, Zheng D, Zou K, et al. Plasma lactate as a marker of metabolic health: Implications of elevated lactate for impairment of aerobic metabolism in the metabolic syndrome. Surgery. 2019;**166**:861-866. DOI: 10.1016/j.surg.2019.04.017

[91] Juraschek SP, Selvin E, Miller ER, Brancati FL, Young JH. Plasma lactate and diabetes risk in 8045 participants of the atherosclerosis risk in communities study. Annals of Epidemiology. 2013;**23**:791-796.e4. DOI: 10.1016/j.annepidem.2013.09.005

[92] Zou K, Turner K, Zheng D, Hinkley JM, Kugler BA, Hornby PJ, et al. Impaired glucose partitioning in primary myotubes from severely obese women with type 2 diabetes. American Journal of Physiology-Cell Physiology. 2020;**319**:C1011-C1019. DOI: 10.1152/ajpcell.00157.2020

[93] Das DK, Graham ZA, Cardozo CP. Myokines in skeletal muscle physiology and metabolism: Recent advances and future perspectives. Acta Physiologica. 2020;**228**:e13367. DOI: 10.1111/apha.13367

[94] Garneau L, Aguer C. Role of myokines in the development of skeletal muscle insulin resistance and related metabolic defects in type 2 diabetes. Diabetes & Metabolism. 2019;**45**:505-516. DOI: 10.1016/j.diabet.2019.02.006

[95] Son JS, Chae SA, Wang H, Chen Y, Bravo Iniguez A, de Avila JM, et al. Maternal inactivity programs skeletal muscle dysfunction in offspring mice by attenuating apelin signaling and mitochondrial biogenesis. Cell Reports. 2020;**33**:108461. DOI: 10.1016/j.celrep.2020.108461

[96] Zunner BEM, Wachsmuth NB, Eckstein ML, Scherl L, Schierbauer JR, Haupt S, et al. Myokines and resistance training: A narrative review. IJMS. 2022;**23**:3501. DOI: 10.3390/ijms23073501

[97] Piccirillo R. Exercise-induced myokines with therapeutic potential for muscle wasting. Frontiers in Physiology. 2019;**10**:287. DOI: 10.3389/fphys.2019.00287

[98] Carson BP. The potential role of contraction-induced myokines in

the regulation of metabolic function for the prevention and treatment of Type 2 diabetes. Frontiers in Endocrinology. 2017;**8**:97. DOI: 10.3389/fendo.2017.00097

[99] Egan B, Zierath JR. Exercise metabolism and the molecular regulation of skeletal muscle adaptation. Cell Metabolism. 2013;**17**:162-184. DOI: 10.1016/j.cmet.2012.12.012

[100] Hughes DC, Ellefsen S, Baar K. Adaptations to endurance and strength training. Cold Spring Harbor Perspectives in Medicine. 2018;**8**:a029769. DOI: 10.1101/cshperspect.a029769

[101] Pan B, Ge L, Xun Y, Chen Y, Gao C, Han X, et al. Exercise training modalities in patients with type 2 diabetes mellitus: A systematic review and network meta-analysis. International Journal of Behavioral Nutrition and Physical Activity. 2018;**15**:72. DOI: 10.1186/s12966-018-0703-3

Chapter 5

# Mechanical Environment in the Human Umbilical Cord and Its Contribution to the Fetal Circulation

*Yoko Kato*


## Abstract

The fetal blood flow in two arteries and one vein of the human umbilical cord could be influenced by the conditions of the fetal growth and placenta that the evaluation of the blood flow pattern by ultrasound Doppler velocimetry is important. That is, the mechanical environment in the umbilical cord should be kept to maintain the blood flow suitable for good fetus growth. In this chapter, a human umbilical cord model for finite analysis, based on the mechanical and histological characteristics is proposed. Considering that the active force production by hyaluronan, proteoglycan, smooth muscle cells, and myofibroblasts could influence the mechanical environment in the umbilical cord, the computation with the proposed model was carried out in order to evaluate the influence. The changes in the mechanical environment caused by the active force production and their influences on the fetal blood flow through the pressure rise and drop in the arteries of the umbilical cord are introduced.


**Keywords:** human umbilical cord, artery, vein, Wharton's jelly, hyaluronan, proteoglycan, smooth muscle cell, myofibroblast, active force production

## 1. Introduction

The human umbilical cord, connecting the fetus and placenta, conveys fetus blood through two arteries and one vein [1]. While the umbilical cord itself spirals, the artery is accompanying the vein with spirals. The blood flow in the umbilical artery and vein, which ultrasound Doppler velocimetry is generally used to measure, shows different characteristics in pulsation: the artery has pulsation, but the vein, except the regions around the ductus venosus and portal vein, does not [2–6]. The difference in pulsation between the artery and vein has been also indicated by pressure [7]. The blood flow pattern could be influenced by the condition of fetal and placenta so that analyses of the flow pattern would be helpful for diagnosis. For example, the pulsation pattern of the blood flow in the artery and vein around the ductus venous and portal vein have been analyzed in pathological aspects [2–6]. In the meantime, the sizes of the umbilical cord, artery, and vein have been reported with some variation [8–14].

Considering the size of the umbilical cord at 40 weeks of gestational age, the diameters of cord, artery, and vein in Ref. [8], whose number of cases was larger than those in [9–14], was 17.8 mm, 4.6 mm, and 9.1 mm at average, respectively, while the length of the cord was more than 50 cm [1]. That is, the blood should travel a long way more than 50 times of the diameter. The distension of the artery and vein of the umbilical cord [15] would contribute to keeping the proper blood flow patterns in the artery and vein, necessary for fetal growth. In numerical analyses, the influence of the umbilical cord's coiling [16] and pressure drop [17] on the blood flow in the artery and vein, and that of arterial pressure pulse on the flow in the vein [18] have been reported. The mechanical environment in the umbilical cord would be arranged as keeping the shapes of the blood vessels, but the investigation has been barely carried out.

The human umbilical artery and vein show the characteristics different from major blood vessels in the body, including large and active endothelial layers [1, 19]. Moreover, the artery has shown two distinctive smooth muscle layers: inner layer, loosely arranged cells with abundant ground substance; outer layer, circularly arranged cells [20]. While myosin and vimentin have been found in both two layers, only the outer layer has indicated desmin [21]. These two blood vessels are covered with Wharton's jelly, whose college fiber has shown the network with canalicular-like structure, and cavernous and perivascular spaces (stromal cleft), which would be helpful for diffusion [22, 23]. Considering the control of the mechanical environment in the umbilical cord, it has been pointed out the contribution of hyaluronan and proteoglycan to pressure control [24], and myofibroblasts, which show active contraction [25, 26].

The mechanical properties of the human umbilical cord and blood vessels have been reported [27–29]. Considering the limitation of the range of the blood pressure in the arteries and vein [7], and nonlinearity in the stress-strain relationship [27–29], the elasticity in the limited range would be proper to estimate the mechanical environment in the umbilical cord. Given that the stress distribution at blood vessel walls would be homogeneous at physiological pressures [30], the assumption that the stress distributions at the umbilical artery and vein would be homogeneous at the average pressure could be made.

In this chapter, a computational model of the human umbilical cord is proposed in order to estimate the mechanical environment. Influence of the change in blood pressure, active force production in smooth muscle cells, myofibroblasts, hyaluronan, and proteoglycan on the mechanical environment and its relation to the fetus's blood flow is shown.

## 2. Computational model of the human umbilical cord

The computational model of the human umbilical cord has been developed on the finite element analysis (FEA) software, COMSOL Multiphysics® ver.6 (COMSOL, Inc. MA). The length of the umbilical cord is longer than 50 times of its diameter so that the cross section, whose normal vector was the axial direction of the umbilical cord, was modeled and analyzed as the representative of the umbilical cord. The analysis has been carried out two-dimensionally, as a plane strain problem.

### 2.1 Spatial arrangement and constraint

The spatial arrangement and size of each component are shown in **Figure 1** and **Table 1**, respectively. The blood vessel is composed of three layers: *Tunica Intima*,

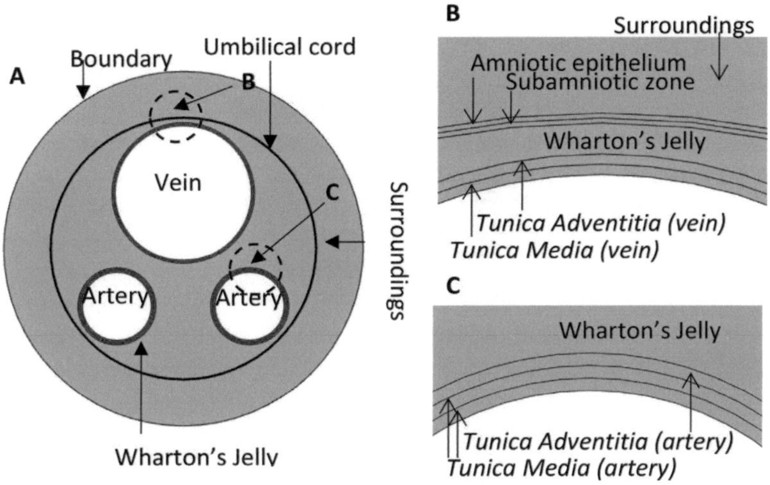


**Figure 1.**
*Components and spatial arrangement in the computational model of the human umbilical cord. A, the entire image of the model; B and C, the vicinities of the vein and artery, respectively.*

| Parameter | Category | Value [mm] | References and comment |
|---|---|---|---|
| Diameter | Cord (outer) | 17.8 | Barbieri C et al. [8] |
| | Artery (inner) | 4.6 | Barbieri C et al. [8] |
| | Vein (inner) | 9.1 | Barbieri C et al. [8] |
| | Boundary | 24.0 | — |
| Thickness | Amniotic epithelium | 0.5 | — |
| | Subamniotic zone | 0.5 | — |
| | Artery | 0.3 | *Tunica Media*, 0.2 mm (two layers); *Tunica Adventitia*, 0.1 mm. |
| | Vein | 0.2 | *Tunica Media*, 0.1 mm; *Tunica Adventitia*, 0.1 mm. |
| Distance | Between the centers of the blood vessels | 8.84 | — |
| | Between the umbilical cord (outer) and the blood vessels (outer) | 0.4 | — |

**Table 1.**
*Sizes of the human umbilical cord model.*

*Tunica Media*, and *Tunica Adventitia*. The intima is composed of a single layer of endothelial cells, and the adventitia shows a sparse distribution of smooth muscle cells without a clear boundary [19] so that the distinctive two layers of smooth muscle, an inner layer with loosely arranged smooth muscle cells and abundant ground substance, and an outer layer with circularly arranged smooth muscle cells [20], was categorized into *Tunica Media* in this study. The diameter of the umbilical cord, and the inner diameters of the artery and vein were the average values *in vivo* at 40 weeks of gestational age in [8], whose number of cases was larger than other reports [9–14].

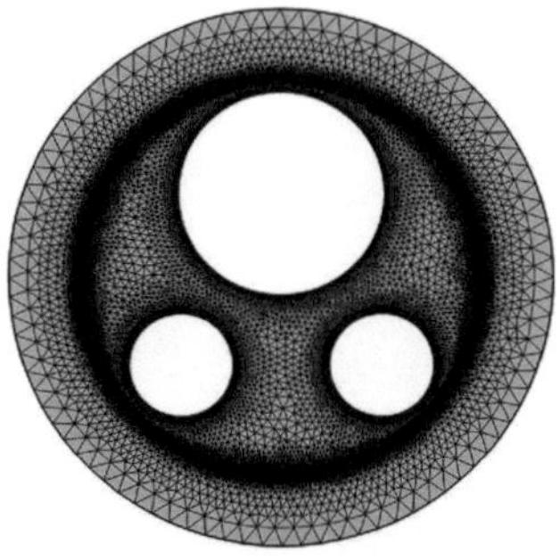

**Figure 2.**
*Finite element model of the human umbilical cord with triangular mesh (the number of elements, 29, 786).*

"Surroundings" and "Boundary" in the model are corresponding to the surroundings of the umbilical cord and limitations in the displacement of the umbilical cord, whose size was about 1.3 times of the umbilical cord's diameter. The thickness values of the amniotic epithelium, subamniotic zone, and blood vessels have been hardly measured *in vivo* so that each thickness was decided as follows: amniotic epithelium and subamniotic zone, less than 5% of the umbilical cord diameter (0.5 mm); artery and vein, only the layers of smooth muscle cells were modeled, and the thickness in each layer was set as 0.1 mm. The center positions of these blood vessels formed an equilateral triangle, whose sides were equally 8.84 mm. All the blood vessels were equally apart from the umbilical cord at the same distance: at the outer diameter, 0.4 mm. **Figure 2** shows the finite element model of the umbilical cord with triangular meshes (the number of elements, 29, 786). The fixation was set on the region, "boundary."

## 2.2 Mechanical properties

The arterial and venous pressure *in vivo* has been reported as 88 mmHg and 41 mmHg on average, respectively [7]. While the venous pressure has hardly shown pulsation, the pressure pulsation in the artery, 12 mmHg, has been observed [7]. The size of each component of the model was based on the measurement *in vivo* so that all the shapes would be at the average pressures in the blood vessels. Given that the stress distribution would be homogeneous at the average pressure [30], the change in stress distribution, caused by the pressure rise and drop (12 mmHg (1.6 kPa)), was evaluated. The pressure in the vein was maintained at 0 Pa because of no pulsation.

Reference [28] has shown the mechanical properties of the umbilical vein and Wharton's jelly with two elastic moduli at high and low stress. Because the removal of the amniotic epithelium has not been mentioned, the results of Wharton's jelly would be those of the umbilical cord without the blood vessel. Also, the description of *Tunica adventitia*, which is difficult to separate properly from the surrounding tissue in general, has not been found so that the sample would include *Tunica media* at least. The stress ($\sigma$) at a thin-walled cylinder caused by the load of internal pressure (P) is calculated by the following equation:

$$\sigma = \frac{Pr}{t} \tag{1}$$

where r and t are the radius and thickness of the cylinder, respectively. When the radius, thickness (*Tunica Media* only), and average pressure at the vein were applied to Eq. (1), the stress was more than 0.1 MPa, which was corresponding to the elastic modulus at high stress [28]. Considering that the surrounding tissues would be also at the high stress, the elastic moduli in *Tunica Media* of the vein and amniotic epithelium were set as 2.36 MPa and 11.1 MPa, respectively as **Table 2**, the list of the mechanical property in each component, shows. While the inner layer of the media in the artery was half of that in the media in the vein (1.18 MPa), the other layers around the blood vessels were set as 2.36 MPa. Considering that blood vessel walls would be incompressible in general, Poisson's ratio was set as 0.4999. Because vimentin, desmin, and α- and γ- actin have been found in the subamniotic zone as well as the layers of the blood vessel, the mechanical properties were set as those in the layers. The components of Wharton's jelly, hyaluronan and proteoglycan, contributing to diffusion, would show its compressibility so that Poisson's ratio was set as 0.1. Supposing that the elastic modulus of Wharton's jelly would be between those of the vein and amniotic epithelium, the lower one, corresponding to that of the vein, was set as that of Wharton's jelly. Plenty of fibers observed in amniotic epithelium [23] would hardly show incompressibility so Poisson's ratio was set as 0.3. Given that the umbilical cord could move freely, the elastic modulus of "Surroundings," corresponding to the surroundings of the umbilical cord, was set as 0.1% of that in the layer of the blood vessel. Also, Poisson's ratio of "Surroundings" was set as 0.4.

The active force productions in the layers of the blood vessels, Wharton's jelly, and subamniotic zone, in each model, are shown in **Table 3**. The magnitude of the force generated by the layers of the blood vessels were two types: one was twice of the other. The force direction was set as the opposite to the pressure in the artery. For evaluating the influence of the layers of the blood vessels and others, the force was 0 Pa (negative) at part of the models: Model A, all the force productions were active; Model B, all the force productions were active and the magnitude was twice of those in Model A; Model C, the force productions at the layers of the blood vessels were active; Model D, the force productions at Wharton's jelly and subamniotic zone were active; Model E, no force production.

| Component | | Elastic modulus [MPa] | Poisson's ratio |
|---|---|---|---|
| Artery | TM (inner) | 1.18 | 0.4999 |
| | TM (outer) | 2.36 | 0.4999 |
| | TA | 2.36 | 0.4999 |
| Vein | TM | 2.36 | 0.4999 |
| | TA | 2.36 | 0.4999 |
| Subamniotic zone | — | 2.36 | 0.4999 |
| Wharton's jelly | — | 2.36 | 0.1 |
| Amniotic epithelium | — | 11.1 | 0.3 |
| Surroundings | — | $2.36 \times 10^{-4}$ | 0.4 |

*TM, Tunica Media; TA, Tunica Adventitia.*

**Table 2.**
*Mechanical properties of the human umbilical cord model.*

| Model | | Active force production (pressure) [Pa] | | | | | | | | |
|---|---|---|---|---|---|---|---|---|---|---|
| | | Blood vessel wall | | | | Subamniotic zone | | Wharton's jelly | | |
| | | Artery | | | Vein | Arterial side | Venous side | Arterial side | Venous side |
| | | TM | | TA | TM & TA | | | | |
| | | inner | outer | | | | | | |
| Pressure rise | A | −160 | −320 | −160 | 160 | −1.6 | 1.6 | −0.8 | 0.8 |
| | B | −320 | −640 | −320 | 320 | −3.2 | 3.2 | −1.6 | 1.6 |
| | C | −160 | −320 | −160 | 160 | 0 | 0 | 0 | 0 |
| | D | 0 | 0 | 0 | 0 | −1.6 | 1.6 | −0.8 | 0.8 |
| | E | 0 | 0 | 0 | 0 | 0 | 0 | 0 | 0 |
| Pressure drop | A | 160 | 320 | 160 | −160 | 1.6 | −1.6 | 0.8 | −0.8 |
| | B | 320 | 640 | 320 | −320 | 3.2 | −3.2 | 1.6 | −1.6 |
| | C | 160 | 320 | 160 | −160 | 0 | 0 | 0 | 0 |
| | D | 0 | 0 | 0 | 0 | 1.6 | −1.6 | 0.8 | −0.8 |
| | E | 0 | 0 | 0 | 0 | 0 | 0 | 0 | 0 |

*TM, Tunica Media; TA, Tunica Adventitia.*

**Table 3.**
*Active force produced in the components. The plus and negative signs are corresponding to the directions of the pressure, outer and inner directions, respectively.*

### 2.3 Mechanical environment

The mechanical environment in the human umbilical cord model was evaluated by von Mises stress ($\sigma_{vm}$) (equivalent stress), described as below:

$$\sigma_{VM} = \frac{1}{\sqrt{2}}\left\{(\sigma_1 - \sigma_2)^2 + (\sigma_2 - \sigma_3)^2 + (\sigma_3 - \sigma_1)^2\right\}^{1/2} \tag{2}$$

where $\sigma_1$, $\sigma_2$, and $\sigma_3$ are three principal stresses. When $\sigma_{vm}$ is equal to the yield stress of a material, the elastic deformation is changed to plastic one. $\sigma_{vm}$ was used as a parameter that estimates how severe the mechanical environment is.

## 3. Mechanical environment in the human umbilical cord

### 3.1 Pressure rise and drop in the arteries

**Figure 3** shows the distribution of von Mises stress ($\sigma_{vm}$) in the umbilical cord model at the pressure rise in the arteries (1.6 kPa). In Models A, and B, where all the components, the layers of the blood vessels, Wharton's jelly, and subamniotic zone, produced active forces, the shapes of the arteries and veins were kept circular. Comparing Model B with Model A, the region for higher $\sigma_{vm}$ around the vein became larger while the region around the arteries reduced. In Models C, D, and E, whose shapes of the blood vessels seemed not circular, higher $\sigma_{vm}$ in the region around the

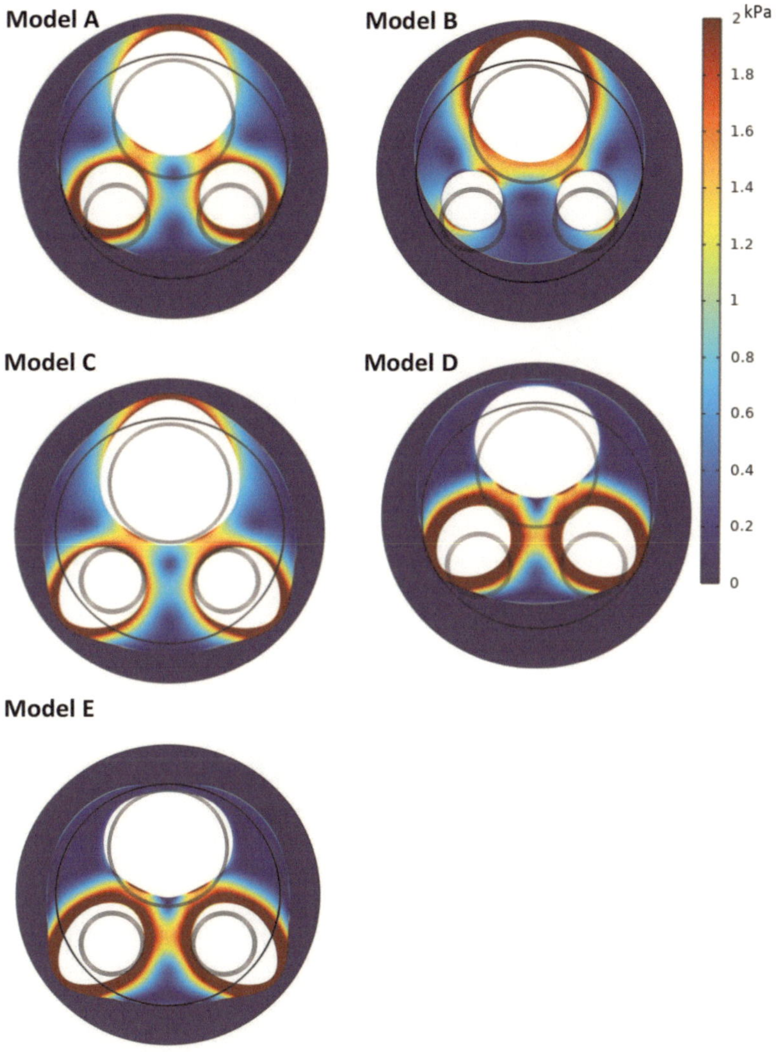


**Figure 3.**
*von Mises stress distribution at the pressure rise in the arteries (1.6 kPa). The black solid line shows the shape before pressure rise. Active force production in each model, indicated in* ***Table 3****, is as follows: Model A, in all the components; Model B, in all the components, twice as large as that in A; Model C, in all the layers around the blood vessels; Model D, in Wharton's jelly and subamniotic zone; E, in no component.*

arteries became larger. **Figure 4** shows the distribution of $\sigma_{vm}$ in detail: $\sigma_{vm}$ along the lines in the umbilical cord, depicted in **Figure 3**, is indicated. All the models indicated that the peak of $\sigma_{vm}$ at the artery and vein sides appeared around the amniotic epithelium in all the lines except Line b-b' at the artery side in the models except Model B. Considering that Line b-b' was passing through the region close to the artery and vein, which would be influenced largely by the pressure rise and active force productions, increase in $\sigma_{vm}$ would be reasonable and could be prevented by an increase in the magnitude of the active force. In the meantime, the peak at the artery side of Line b-b' was much smaller than other peaks so that the regions around the blood vessels would keep smaller than those around the amniotic epithelium. The peak of $\sigma_{vm}$ at Models B (vein side), and D and E (artery side) was larger than that in

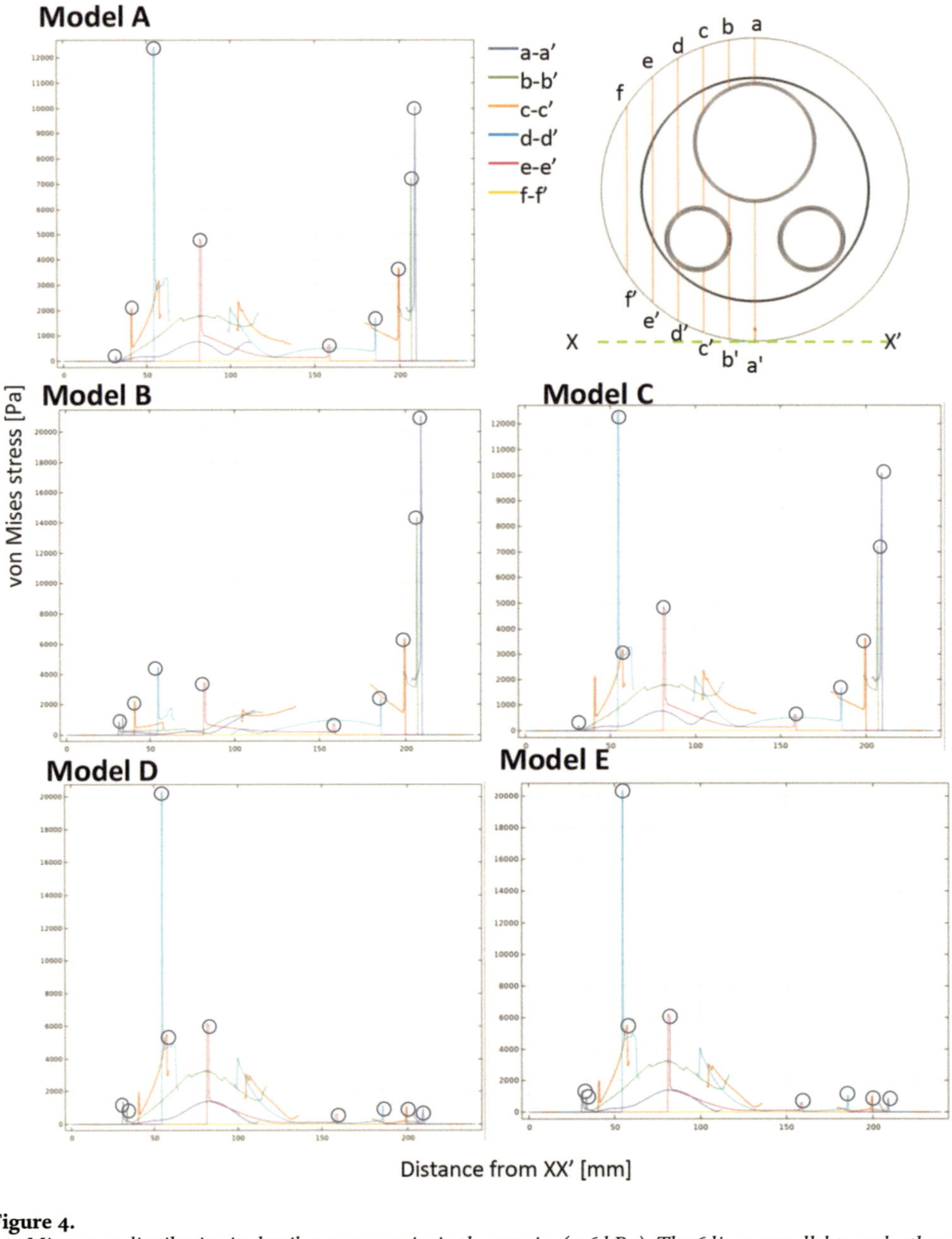


**Figure 4.**
*von Mises stress distribution in detail at pressure rise in the arteries (1.6 kPa). The 6 lines, parallel to each other at the space interval of 0.2 mm from the center to the surroundings (the top of the right side.) were set to examine the stress distribution. The stress along the line in each model is indicated with the circles, corresponding to the peak at the artery and vein sides.*

Models A and C. The magnitude of the active force production at Model B would be too large. And the force produced by the layers of the blood vessels would be necessary to modulate the stress distribution in the umbilical cord.

**Figure 5** shows the distribution of von Mises stress ($\sigma_{vm}$) in the umbilical cord model at the pressure drop in the arteries (1.6 kPa). Models A and B, where the active forces were produced at all the components, kept the shape of the blood vessels circular. While Model B had the larger region around the vein for higher $\sigma_{vm}$ than

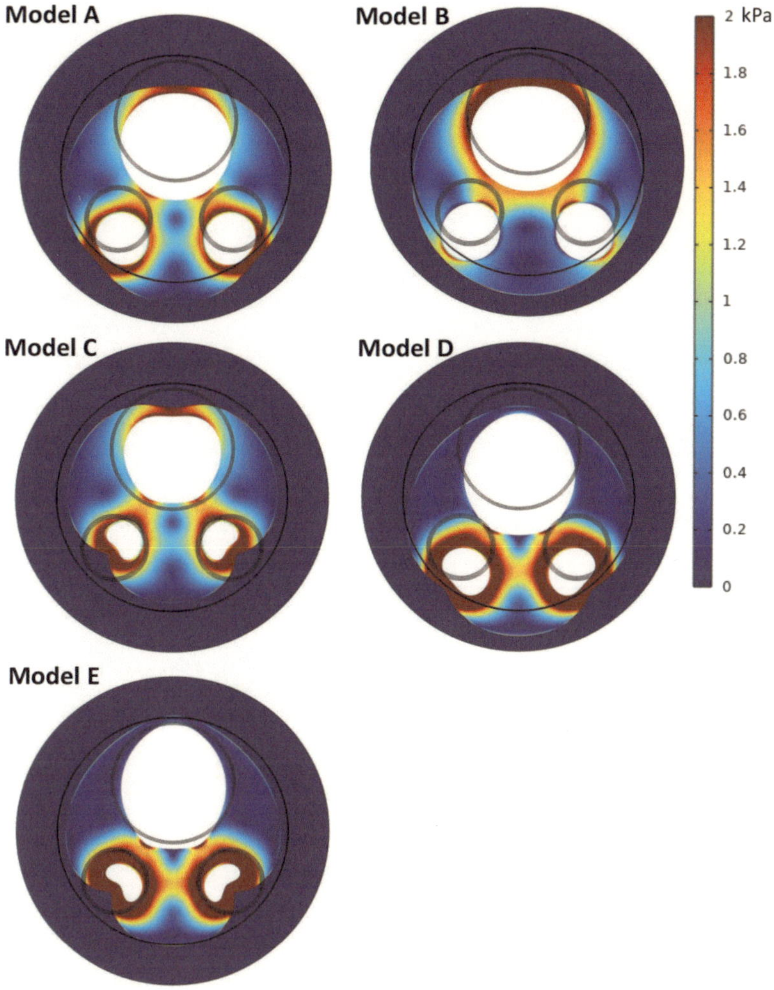


**Figure 5.**
*von Mises stress distribution at the pressure drop in the arteries (1.6 kPa). The black solid line shows the shape before pressure drop. Active force production in each model, indicated in* ***Table*** *3, is as follows: Model A, in all the components; Model B, in all the components, twice as large as that in A; Model C, in all the layers around the blood vessels; Model D, in Wharton's jelly and subamniotic zone; E, in no component.*

Model A, the regions around the arteries for higher $\sigma_{vm}$ in Model B were smaller than those in Model A. The circular shapes of the blood vessels have been hardly kept in Models C, D, and E, with the larger regions around the arteries for higher $\sigma_{vm}$. These characteristics of the shapes of the blood vessels and distribution pattern of $\sigma_{vm}$ were similar to those in pressure rise as **Figures 3** and **5** show although Models C, D, and E caused the collapses of the arteries and umbilical cord, which were not observed in those models at the pressure rise. **Figure 6** shows the $\sigma_{vm}$ along the lines, which were set as the case of pressure rise in **Figure 4**. The characteristics of all the graphs in **Figure 6** agreed with those in **Figure 4** because the pressures rise and drop had the same magnitude with different directions, and $\sigma_{vm}$ is the function of the difference between the principal stresses as Eq. (2) shows. Hence, through the change in the arterial pressure, the stress around the blood vessels would be kept much lower than that around the amniotic epithelium.

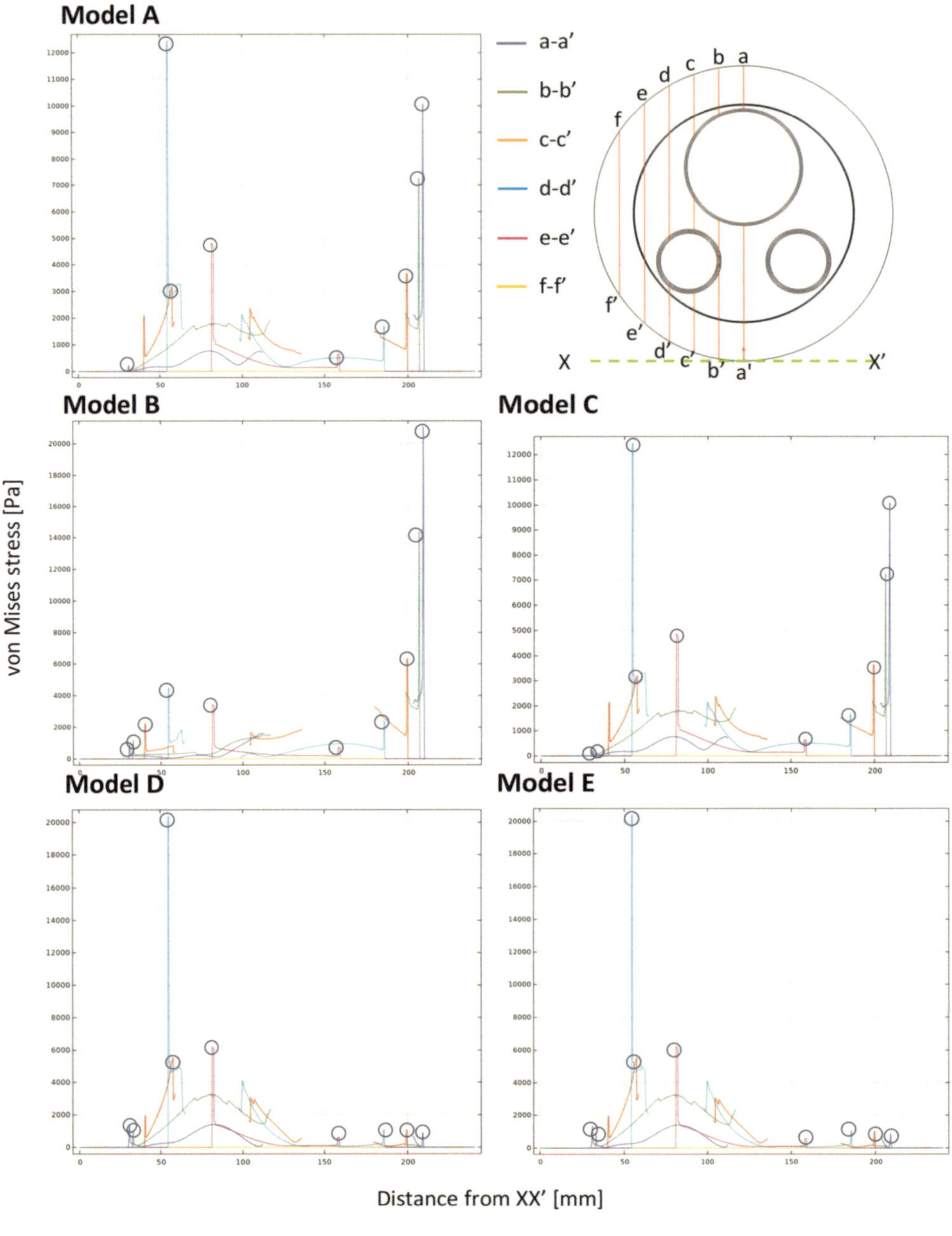


**Figure 6.**
*von Mises stress distribution in detail at pressure drop in the arteries (1.6 kPa). The 6 lines, parallel to each other at the space interval of 0.2 mm from the center to the surroundings (the top of the right side.) were set to examine the stress distribution. The stress along the line in each model is indicated with the circles, corresponding to the peak at the artery and vein sides.*

### 3.2 Mechanical environment and blood flow in the umbilical cord

The $\sigma_{vm}$ around the blood vessels (< 6 kPa) was kept much lower than that around the amniotic epithelium (> 12 kPa) when the pressure in the arteries and the active force production was changed. Considering that the adaptations of the blood vessels and the surrounding tissue to change in the mechanical environment could cause changes in their shapes and structures, the control of the mechanical environment would be effective to keep the shapes and structures of these components in the umbilical cord. Also, considering the adaptation and damage in the amniotic epithelium might be necessary. In the meantime, the shape of the blood vessels would be hardly kept unless the active forces were produced by all the components. The shape of the blood vessel would directly influence the blood flow pattern and cause change in wall shear stress, which could damage the blood vessel function and structure. Also, the collapse of the umbilical cord at the pressure drop with the active forces, which were produced partially, could damage its tissue structure. Hence, the active force productions at all the components would be necessary to maintain the proper blood flow in the umbilical blood vessels and avoid the damage to the tissue of the umbilical cord.

## 4. Conclusion

The human umbilical cord model for finite element analysis, based on the mechanical and histological characteristics, has been developed. The influence of the active force productions by hyaluronan, proteoglycan, smooth muscle cells, and myofibroblasts on the stress distribution in the umbilical cord was evaluated. As a result, the active forces produced by all the components would be necessary to maintain the blood flow properly.

## Acknowledgements

This work was supported by Grant for Individual Research of Tohoku-Gakuin in 2021.

## Conflict of interest

The author declares no conflict of interest.

## Author details

Yoko Kato
Faculty of Engineering, Tohoku Gakuin University, Miyagi, Japan

*Address all correspondence to: ykato@mail.tohoku-gakuin.ac.jp

## References

[1] Kaplan CG. Anatomy and pathology of the umbilical cord. In: Baergen RN, Burton GJ, Kaplan CG, editors. Benirschkes's Pathology of the Human Placenta. 7th ed. Cham: Springer; 2022. pp. 345-402. DOI: 10.1007/978-3-030-84725-8_16

[2] Todros T, Piccoli E, Rolfo A, Cardaropoli S, Guito C, Gaglioti P, et al. Review: Feto-placental vascularization: A multifaceted approach. Placenta. 2011; **Suppl 2**:S165-S169. DOI: 10.1016/j.placenta.2010.12.020

[3] Sutton MS, Theard MA, Bhatia SJ, Plappert T, Saltzman DH, Doubilet P. Changes in placental blood flow in the normal human fetus with gestational age. Pediatric Research. 1990;**28**(4): 383-387. DOI: 10.1203/00006450-199010000-00016

[4] Kiserud T. The ductus venosus. Seminars in Perinatology. 2001;**25**(1): 11-20. DOI: 10.1053/sper.2001.22896

[5] Braga M, Moleiro ML, Guedes-Martins LG. Clinical significance of ductus venosus waveform as generated by pressure-volume changes in the fetal heart. Current Cardiology Reviews. 2019;**15**(3):167-176. DOI: 10.2174/1573403X15666190115142303

[6] Bellotti M, Pennati G, Gasperi CD, Bozzo M, Battaglia FC, Ferrazzi E. Simultaneous measurement of umbilical venous, fetal hepatic, and ductus venosus blood flow in growth-restricted human fetuses. American Journal of Obstetrics and Gynecology. 2004; **190**(5):1347-1358. DOI: 10.1016/j.ajog.2003.11.018

[7] Malpas P, Symonds EM. Arterial and venous pressure in the human umbilical cord. American Journal of Obstetrics and Gynecology. 1967;**98**(2):261-265. DOI: 10.1016/s0002-9378(16)34596-3

[8] Barbieri C, Cecatti JG, Surita FG, Marussi EF, Costa JV. Sonographic measurement of the umbilical cord area and the diameters of its vessels during pregnancy. Journal of Obstetrics and Gynaecology. 2012;**32**:230-236. DOI: 10.3109/01443615.2011.647129

[9] Ghezzi F, Raio L, Naro ED, Franchi M, Balestereri D, D'Addario V. Normogram of Wharton's jelly as depicted in the sonographic cross section of the umbilical cord. Ultrasound in Obstetrics & Gynecology. 2001;**18**(2): 121-125. DOI: 10.1046/j.1469-0705.2001.00468.x

[10] Raio L, Ghezzi F, Naro ED, Gomez R, Franchi M, Mazor M, et al. Sonographic measurement of the umbilical cord and fetal anthropometric parameters. European journal of obstetrics, gynecology, and reproductive biology. 1999;**83**(2):131-135. DOI: 10.1016/s0301-2115(98)00314-5

[11] Proctor KL, Fitzgerald B, Whittle WL, Mokhtari N, Lee E, Machin G, et al. Umbilical cord diameter percentile curves and their correlation to birth weight and placental pathology. Placenta. 2013;**34**(1):62-66. DOI: 10.1016/j.placenta.2012.10.015

[12] Rostamzadeh S, Kalantari M, Shahrizi M, Shakiba M. Sonographic measurement of the umbilical cord and its vessel and their relation with fetal anthropometric measurements. Iranian Journal of Radiology. 2015;**12**(3):e12230. DOI: 10.5812/iranjradiol.12230v2

[13] Togni FA, Júnior EA, Vasques FAP, Moron AF, Torloni MR, Nardozza LMM.

The cross-section area of umbilical cord components in normal pregnancy. International Journal of Gynecology and Obstetrics. 2007;**96**(3):156-161. DOI: 10.1016/j.ijgo.2006.10.003

[14] Weissman A, Jakobi P. Sonographic measurements of the umbilical cord in pregnancies complicated by gestational diabetes. Journal of Ultrasound in Medicine. 1997;**16**(10):691-694. DOI: 10.7863/jum.1997.16.10.691

[15] Reynolds SRM. The proportion of Wharton's jelly in the umbilical cord in relation to distention of the umbilical arteries and vein, with observations on the folds of Hoboken. The Anatomical Record. 1952;**113**(3):365-377. DOI: 10.1002/ar.1091130309

[16] Wilke DJ, Denier JP, Khong TY, Mattner TW. Pressure and flow in the umbilical cord. Journal of Biomechanics. 2018;**79**:78-87. DOI: 10.1016/j.jbiomech.2018.07.044

[17] Wilke DJ, Denier JP, Khong TY, Mattner TW. Estimating umbilical cord flow resistance from measurements of the whole cord. Placenta. 2021;**103**: 180-187. DOI: 10.1016/j.placenta.2020.09.066

[18] Waters SL, Guiot C. Flow in an elastic tube subject to prescribed forcing: A model of umbilical venous flow. Computational and Mathematical Methods in Medicine. 2001;**3**:287-298. DOI: 10.1080/10273660108833081

[19] Sexton AJ, Turmaine M, Cai WQ, Burnstock G. A study of the ultrastructure of developing human umbilical vessels. Journal of Anatomy. 1996;**188**:75-88

[20] Mayer WW, Rumpelt HJ, Yao AC, Lind J. Structure and closure mechanism of the human umbilical artery. European Journal of Pediatrics. 1978;**128**:247-259. DOI: 10.1007/BF00445610

[21] Nanaev AK, Shirinsky VP, Birukov KG. Immunofluorescent study of heterogeneity in smooth muscle cells of human fetal vessels using antibodies to myosin, desmin, and vimentin. Cell and Tissue Research. 1991;**266**:535-540. DOI: 10.1007/BF00318595

[22] Vizza E, Correr S, Goranova V, Heyn R, Muglia U, Papagianni V. The collagen fibrils arrangement in the Wharton's jelly of full-term human umbilical cord. Italian Journal of Anatomy and Embryology. 1995;**100** (Suppl 1):495-501.

[23] Vizza E, Correr S, Goranova V, Heyn R, Angelucci PA, Forleo R, et al. The collagen skeleton of the human umbilical cord at term. A scanning electron microscopy study after 2N-NAOH maceration. Reproduction, Fertility, and Development. 1996;**8**: 885-894. DOI: 10.1071/rd9960885

[24] Meyer FA. Wharton's jelly of the umbilical cord. In: Comper WD, editor. Exracellular Matrix. Vol. 1. The Netherlands: Harwood Academic Publishers; 1996. pp. 443-456

[25] Takechi K, Kuwabara Y, Mizuno M. Ultrastructural and immunohistochemical studies of Wharton's jelly umbilical cord. Placenta. 1993;**14**:235-245. DOI: 10.1016/s0143-4004(05)80264-4

[26] Nanaev AK, Kohnen G, Milovanov AP, Domogatsky SP, Kaufmann P. Stromal differentiation and architecture of the human umbilical cord. Placenta. 1997;**18**:53-64. DOI: 10.1016/s0143-4004(97)90071-0

[27] Ghosh KG, Ghosh SN, Gupta AB. Tensile properties of human umbilical

cord. The Indian Journal of Medical Research. 1984;**79**:538-541

[28] Pennati G. Biomechanical properties of the human umbilical cord. Biorheology. 2001;**38**:355-366

[29] Nye KS, Esplin MS, Monson KL. Umbilical cord artery mechanical properties at various gestational ages. American Journal of Perinatology. 2015; **32**(3):263-270. DOI: 10.1055/s-0034-1383850

[30] Takamizawa K, Hayashi K. Strain energy density function and uniform strain hypothesis for arterial mechanics. Journal of Biomechanics. 1987;**20**(1): 7-17. DOI: 10.1016/0021-9290(87)90262-4

## Chapter 6

# Use of CPAP in Premature Babies

*Prema Subramaniam*


## Abstract

Respiratory distress syndrome (RDS) is the most common respiratory disorder of preterm infants and is a major course of neonatal mortality and morbidity. The combined use of antenatal steroids and early continuous positive airway pressure (CPAP) are considered the gold standard for the prevention and treatment of RDS in the preterm infant. CPAP used in the spontaneous breathing neonate maintains adequate functional residual capacity within the alveoli to prevent atelectasis and support gas exchange CPAP is most commonly delivered using bi-nasal short prongs or a nasal mask. Pressure is generated using a variety of devices. CPAP is generally well tolerated, in part because infants are preferential or "obligatory nasal breathers". CPAP has revolutionised the outcome in premature babies by reducing the need for mechanical ventilation and the use of surfactant. Prophylactic or early CPAP in the delivery room reduces the need for surfactant and mechanical ventilation by nearly 50%. CPAP is an attractive option for supporting neonates with respiratory distress, because it preserves spontaneous breathing, does not require endotracheal intubation, and may result in less lung injury than mechanical ventilation.


**Keywords:** CPAP, RDS, prematurity, reduction in mortality and morbidity, surfactant

## 1. Introduction

Globally around 2.4 million newborns died in 2020 of which 75% of neonatal deaths occur within the first week of life. In 2017 most neonatal deaths occurred as a result of either preterm birth, intrapartum complications such as birth asphyxia or failing to breath, infections and/or lethal congenital malformations [1].

Respiratory distress syndrome (RDS) in the newborn is one of the major causes of neonatal mortality and morbidity. RDS is due to a lack of surfactant in the lungs of the preterm baby and this usually develops in the first 24 h of life. Positive pressure ventilation has been found to be an effective form of treatment for this condition [2].

In women at risk of preterm birth treatment the use of antenatal corticosteroids has been proven to reduce perinatal and neonatal death, RDS and Intraventricular haemorrhages (IVH) [3]. The combined use of antenatal steroids and early continuous positive airway pressure (CPAP) are considered the gold standard for the prevention and treatment of RDS in the preterm infant [4, 5].

## 2. CPAP

### 2.1 What is nasal CPAP?

Nasal continuous airway pressure (CPAP) is a non-invasive form of respiratory support for the spontaneously breathing infant with lung disease. In this situation CPAP provides a constant distending pressure during both the inhalation and expiration phases thereby reducing the need for intubation and mechanical ventilation [6].

CPAP imitates the natural physiologic reflex called "grunting," which is forced expiration against a closed glottis that occurs with infants with poor lung compliance and low end-expiratory volume who uses this physiological mechanism to try to maintain a higher end expiratory volume [7].

The infants tongue and soft palate forms an anatomic seal thereby maintaining the CPAP pressure in the babies lungs [8].

CPAP maintains functional residual capacity (FRC) and supports gas exchange in the neonatal lungs thereby reducing the incidence of apnoea, improves the work of breathing and reduces lung damage [9].

CPAP was first used to support the breathing of preterm infants in 1971 [10]. Gregory used Endotracheal tubes for his CPAP study in 20 infants weighing between 930 and 3800 g. All these infants had severe RDS and were breathing spontaneously. Gregory used pressures up to 12 mmHg via the ETT in 18 of the infants and for the other 2 infants he used a pressure chamber placed around the infants head. He noted that increasing the PEEP (positive end expiratory pressure) caused a reduction in the minute ventilation. However there was not much change in the babies pH, $CO_2$ tension, blood pressure or lung compliance.

### 2.2 How does CPAP benefit infants with RDS?

The surfactant deficiency in RDS causes collapse of the terminal airways in the babies lungs leading to a reduction in the functional residual capacity. This results in an increase in the ventilation-perfusion mismatch and thereby an increase in the work of breathing [11].

CPAP reduces upper airway obstruction by the decrease in pulmonary vascular resistance and increasing the thoracic gas volume [12–14].

CPAP also decreases left to right shunting by increasing right ventricular output while not significantly affecting the left ventricular output and pulmonary vascular resistance [15].

CPAP also produces a rise in Pa02 (with no significant change in PCO2) and maintains the Positive End Expiratory Pressure (PEEP) thereby reducing atelectasis, increasing the surface area of the alveolus and thereby an improvement in the ventilation-perfusion mismatch [16, 17]. The rise in Pa02 and the resulting regulation in both rate and dept. of respiration generally results in a cessation of grunting with 15 min of commencing CPAP. CPAP thereby improves the infants ability to cope with increasing respiratory loads through the Hering-Breuer reflex [18].

CPAP in most instances is applied at pressures between 4 and 6 cm $H_2O$ however, in infants with poor lung compliance, CPAP of pressures from 8 to 10 cm $H_2O$ have been used. The higher pressures might result in overdistension that affects gas exchange and damage to the terminal airways may result in pneumothorax. It is uncertain what the optimum CPAP levels should be as this varies with the age of the infant and the severity of RDS [19].

### 2.3 Use of CPAP in neonates

CPAP is commonly used in neonates with the following conditions:

1. RDS

   Prophylactic CPAP i.e. CPAP started immediately after delivery in preterm or low birth weight infant or within the first 15 min of life (before the onset of respiratory disease) has been shown to reduce the incidence of BPD (broncho-pulmonary disease), the combined outcome of death or BPD, and the need for mechanical ventilation [20, 21].
   In preterm or low birth weight infants with established respiratory distress, CPAP reduces the incidence of respiratory failure, the use of mechanical ventilation and mortality however there is an increased rate of pneumothorax compared to spontaneous breathing with supplemental oxygen [3].

2. Post extubation

   NCPAP can also be used as "step-down" therapy to provide respiratory support following extubation after mechanical ventilation. These infants have a less likelihood of developing respiratory failure and having the need for reintubation and mechanical ventilation. The reason for this may be due to the fact that CPAP maintains lung volumes, causes airflow stimulation of the nasal passage and upper airway and by reducing apnoea in the preterm infant [22, 23].

3. Apnoea

   CPAP decreases both obstructive and a combination of obstructive and central apnoea and prevents hypoxia. Central apnoea by itself is not affected by CPAP. Miller postulated that CPAP reduces upper airway obstruction by splinting the pharyngeal airway [24].

### 2.4 CPAP apparatus

CPAP has two main components: a device to generate pressure and a patient interface used to deliver pressure.

CPAP devices include:

Variable flow devices ie devices that generate CPAP by a jet of blended air delivered by the Infant Flow Driver. This system requires air flows in excess of 8 L/min in order to generate positive end expiratory pressures of 5 cm $H_2O$.

Constant or continuous flow examples of which are bubble CPAP and ventilator CPAP.

With bubble CPAP the PEEP is maintained by immersing the distal end of the expiratory tubing in water. The pressures are determined by the depth of the tubing in the water. For example 5 cm below the surface equals to 5 cm $H_2O$ blended humidified gas oxygen or air is delivered by nasal prongs or nasal masks and as air flows out of the infant via the expiratory tubing it gives its characteristic bubbling [1, 3, 25]. Bubble CPAP is inexpensive and is easy to adapt for newborns [3]; however, if the interface is not well adapted or if there is leakage through the nose or mouth, the PEEP is not guaranteed.

Studies have shown that there is little difference in terms of respiratory rate, heart rate, blood pressure or comfort scores between the use of continuous flow CPAP and variable flow CPAP [8, 26–31].

Many neonatal units use CPAP pressures delivered between 5 and 6 cm $H_2O$. Some units use starting pressures of 8 cm $H_2O$. Elgellab noted that CPAP pressures of 8 cm $H_2O$ improved the thoraco-abdominal synchrony, lowered the respiratory rate and increased the tidal volume of preterm infants with respiratory failure [18].

For preterm infants with poorly compliant lungs, higher CPAP pressures 32 (e.g. 8 cm $H_2O$ may be needed 3 as the first line of support immediately after birth or at the start of the respiratory distress with escalation to intubation and mechanical ventilation if CPAP fails.

## 2.5 CPAP delivery

The most common interfaces for CPAP delivery include:

Short binasal prongs that fits directly into the nostrils or nasal mask. Other interfaces used included single nasal prongs and nasopharyngeal prongs which uses a nasopharyngeal tube (NGT) in which the tip of the tube sits in the nasopharynx thereby bypassing the nasal cavity [32, 33].

Short binasal prongs when compared to single nasal prongs and nasopharyngeal prongs showed that there was a decrease in the babies oxygen requirement and respiratory rate thereby reducing the need for reintubation [23, 34, 35]. Endotracheal tubes are still used to deliver CPAP when the infants have facial anomalies such as bilateral cleft lip and or palate [2].

The problem with binasal prongs however is that it must be fitted snugly which can lead to injury to the nares and nasal septum [35, 36].

With the nasal mask, this is placed over the babies nose and mouth forming a good seal.

When compared to binasal prongs, nasal masks decreased the incidence of moderate-to-severe BPD and the need for surfactant. However there were no differences in mortality or other morbidities [7, 30].

CPAP failure i.e. babies requiring mechanical ventilation while on CPAP is defined when one or more of the following conditions arise: persistent or frequent apnoeic episodes, PaCO2 of $\geq$60 mm Hg (8.3 kPa), FiO2 of $\geq$0.6 to maintain acceptable oxygen saturation. 14% to as high as 40% of infants with respiratory distress who have initially been started on CPAP may need to be intubated and ventilated. CPAP failure was associated with an increased rate of pneumothorax, death, bronchopulmonary dysplasia (BPD) and other morbidities compared with those managed on CPAP alone [37–39].

## 2.6 Contraindications in the use of CPAP in babies

This includes upper airway abnormalities such as choanal atresia, cleft palate and trachea oeophageal fistula.

Babies in shock i.e. cardiovascular instability.

Frequent apnoeic episodes with bradycardia and desaturations.

Respiratory failure PCO2 of >60 mmHg FiO2 > 0.6 to maintain an acceptable O2 saturation.

Congenital diaphragmatic hernia as the gastric distension caused by CPAP can result in further compromise of the organs in the chest.

Complications that can occur with CPAP giving rise to inefficient delivery include [40]

- Kinking of nasopharyngeal tube (in NP CPAP) and/or delivery circuit.
- Obstruction of the binasal nasal prongs with mucus plugging.
- Displacement of the nasal prongs/mask.
- Skin irritation of the face from the securing tapes.
- Pressure necrosis around nostrils and distortion of the nasal septum.
- Pressure necrosis around head/ears due to improperly secured bonnets or CPAP head harnesses.
- Air leaking around the prongs due to the mouth being open which may result in loss of desired pressure and decrease in delivered oxygen concentration.
- Pneumothorax or pneumomediastinum especially in the extremely low birth weight babies.
- Extremely high CPAP levels resulting in a decrease in the venous return and therefore reducing the babies cardiac output.
- Feed intolerance following gastric distension (CPAP belly) as the delivered gas enters the stomach and gastrointestinal tract.

### 2.7 CPAP and surfactant

Studies have shown that in babies with moderate to severe respiratory distress syndrome the combination of nasal continuous positive airway pressure (nCPAP) and a single dose of surfactant reduces the need for intubation and mechanical ventilation [36].

Methods of delivering surfactant to an infant on CPAP include:

INSURE method (INtubation-SURfactant-Extubation), Surfactant administration via thin catheter and Nebulized surfactant [41].

The INSURE method (INtubation-SURfactant-Extubation) is done by intubating the infant, administrating surfactant via the endotracheal tube followed by a short period of mechanical ventilation, extubation and then onto CPAP. This is done at the onset of RDS [42] Stevens suggest that in spontaneously breathing preterm infants with RDS the INSURE method of surfactant administration followed by early extubation to NCPAP is preferable to traditional intubation and surfactant treatment and keeping the baby on the ventilator. INSURE reduces the need for mechanical ventilation. Its also reduces the incidence of pneumothorax and BPD.

Surfactant administration via thin catheter (S-TC) encompasses any method in which a thin catheter, narrower than a standard endotracheal tube (ETT), is passed through the vocal cords to allow surfactant instillation. The most commonly used methods are [43].

A flexible thin catheter and Magill's forceps (Cologne method), as described by Kribs and colleagues [33], flexible thin feeding tube without Magill's forceps (take care method), as described by Kanmaz and colleagues, semi-rigid thin catheter (Hobart method), as described by Dargaville and colleagues [30]; and modifications of the above methods.

Differences of the various methods may be encountered in (1) the pre-medication used, (2) the means of laryngoscopy used, including videolaryngoscopy, (3) the type of catheter, (4) the method used to guide the catheter through the vocal cords, (5) the approach to surfactant delivery (bolus versus infusion, rapid versus slow), (6) the surfactant preparation, (7) the surfactant dose, and (8) the approach to respiratory management before, during, and after the technique, including the type of non-invasive respiratory support used. It is expected that infants are spontaneously breathing, and therefore positive-pressure inflations are not required for surfactant dispersal. Unlike an ETT, a thin catheter is unsuitable for delivery of positive-pressure inflations.

Several different acronyms may be used for the above methods, including:

- MIST (minimally invasive surfactant therapy);
- LISA (less invasive surfactant administration);
- SurE (surfactant without endotracheal tube);
- MISA (minimally invasive surfactant administration); and
- NISA (non-invasive surfactant administration).

Abdel-Latif et al. concluded in his Cochrane review that surfactant therapy via thin catheter (S-TC) compared to surfactant via endotracheal tube (ETT) reduced the incidence of the combined outcome of death or bronchopulmonary dysplasia (BPD) at 36 weeks' postmenstrual age (PMA) [31].

### 2.8 Nebulised surfactant

This method is carried out when Aerosolised surfactant is given to the neonate via a customised vibrating membrane nebuliser positioned between the mask and the bubble nCPAP circuit. Minocchieri et al. showed that nebulised surfactant administered in the first 4 h of life to very and moderately preterm infants with mild RDS may benefit these babies [44]. These findings require confirmation in a adequately powered randomised controlled trial evaluating the benefits of nebulised surfactant in infants with mild to moderate respiratory distress [44].

## 3. Conclusion

In conclusion CPAP is a safe and effective method of noninvasive ventilation in the preterm infant with RDS and it reduces the need for assisted ventilation by almost half, and substantially reduced the use of surfactant. CPAP is a simple and inexpensive form of treatment to implement and hence has implications for use in low- and middle-income countries (LMIC).

## Conflict of interest

The author declares no conflict of interest.

## Author details

Prema Subramaniam
Mount Isa Hospital, Mount Isa, Queensland, Australia

*Address all correspondence to: sprema882yahoo.co.nz

## References

[1] Newborn Mortality: World Health Organization. Fact Sheet. 28 Jan 2022

[2] Ainsworth SB. Pathophysiology of neonatal respiratory distress syndrome: Implications for early treatment strategies treat. Respiratory Medicine. 2005;**4**(6):423-423. DOI: 10.2165/00151829-200504060-00006

[3] Ho JJ, Subramaniam P, Davis PG. Continuous positive airway pressure (CPAP) for respiratory distress in preterm infants. Cochrane Library of Systematic Reviews [Internet]. 15 Oct 2020;**10**(10):CD002271. DOI: 10.1002/14651858.CD002271.pub3

[4] McGoldrick E, Stewart F, Parker R, Dalziel S. Antenatal corticosteroids for accelerating fetal lung maturation for women at risk of preterm birth. Cochrane Data base of Systemic Reviews [Internet]. 2020;(12). DOI: 10.1002/14651858.CD004454.pub4

[5] Roberts D, Brown J, Medley N, Dalziel SR. Antenatal corticosteroids for accelerating fetal lung maturation for women at risk of preterm birth. Cochrane Database of Systematic Reviews. 2017;**3**(3):CD004454. Available from:. DOI: 10.1002/14651858. CD004454.pub3

[6] Subramaniam P, Ho JJ, Davis PG. Prophylactic or very early initiation of continuous positive airway pressure (CPAP) for preterm infants. Cochrane Database of Systematic Reviews [Internet]. 2021;**10**(10):CD001243. DOI: 10.1002/14651858.CD001243.pub4

[7] Gregory GA, Edmunds LH Jr, Kitterman JA, Phibbs RH, Tooley WH. Continuous positive airway pressure and pulmonary and circulatory function after cardiac surgery in infants less than three months of age. Anesthesiology. 1975;**43**(4):426-431

[8] Bhatti A, Khan J, Murki S, Sundaram V, Saini SS, Kumar P. Nasal Jet-CPAP (variable flow) versus Bubble-CPAP in preterm infants with respiratory distress: An open label, randomized controlled trial. Journal of Perinatology. 2015;**35**(11):935-940. DOI: 10.1038/jp.2015.98. Epub 2015 Aug 13

[9] DiBlasi RM. Nasal continuous positive airway pressure (CPAP) for the respiratory care of the newborn infant. Respiratory Care. 2009;**54**(9):1209-1235

[10] Subramaniam P, Ho JJ, Davis PG. Prophylactic nasal continuous positive airway pressure for preventing morbidity and mortality in very preterm infants. Cochrane Neonatal Group, editor. Cochrane Database of Systematic Reviews [Internet]. 2016. DOI: doi.wiley.com/10.1002/14651858.CD001243.pub3

[11] Mukerji A, Wahab MG, Mitra S, Mondal T, Paterson D, Beck J, et al. High continuous positive airway pressure in neonates: A physiological study. Pediatric Pulmonology. 2019;**7**:1039-1044

[12] Gregory GA, Kitterman JA, Phibbs RH, et al. Treatment of the idiopathic respiratory-distress syndrome with continuous positive airway pressure. New England Journal of Medicine. 1971;**284**:1333-1340

[13] Cotton RB, Lindstrom DP, Kanarek KS, Sundell H, Stahlman MT. Effect of positive-end-expiratory-pressure on right ventricular output in lambs with hyaline membrane disease. Acta Paediatrica Scandinavica.

1980;**69**(5):603-606. DOI: 10.1111/j.1651-2227.1980.tb07329.x

[14] Saunders RA, Milner AD, Hopkin IE. The effects of CPAP on lung mechanics and lung volumes in the. Biology of the neonate. 1976;**29**(3-4):178-186. DOI: 10.1159/000240862

[15] Alex CG et al. Effects of continuous positive airway pressure on upper airway and respiratory muscle activity. Journal of Applied Physiology. 1987;**62**:2026-2030

[16] Richardson CP, Jung AL. Effects of continuous positive airway pressure on pulmonary function and blood gases of infants with respiratory distress syndrome. Pediatric Research. 1978;**12**(7):771-774. DOI:10.1203/00006450-197807000-00006

[17] Martin RJ, Nearman HS, Katona PG, Klaus MH. The effect of a low continuous positive airway pressure on the reflex control of respiration in the preterm infant. Journal of Pediatrics. 1977;**90**(6):976-981

[18] Nicolas B, Julie Fierro J, Mukerji A, Wright CJ, Millar D, Kirpalani H. Nasal continuous positive airway pressure levels for the prevention of morbidity and mortality in preterm infants. Cochrane Database of Systematic Reviews [Internet]. 30 Nov 2021. DOI: 10.1002/14651858.CD012778.pub2

[19] Speidel BD, Dunn PM. Effect of continuous positive airway pressure on breathing patterns of infants with respiratory distress syndrome. Lancet. 1975;**i**:302-304

[20] Bamat N, Fierro J, Mukerji A, Wright CJ, Millar D, Kirpalani H. Nasal continuous positive airway pressure levels for the prevention of morbidity and mortality in preterm infants. Cochrane Database of Systematic Reviews. 2021;**11**(11):CD012778. DOI: 10.1002/14651858.CD012778.pub2

[21] Wiswell TE, Srinivasan P. Continuous positive airway pressure. In: Goldsmith JP, Karotkin EH, editors. Assisted Ventilation of the Neonate. 4th ed. Philadelphia: WB Saunders; 2004. pp. 127-147

[22] Davis PG, Henderson-Smart DJ. Nasal continuous positive airway pressure immediately after extubation for preventing morbidity in preterm infants. Cochrane Database of Systematic Reviews [Internet]. 2003;(2):CD000143. DOI: 10.1002/14651858.CD000143

[23] Davis PG, Henderson-Smart DJ. Nasal continuous positive airways pressure immediately after extubation for preventing morbidity in preterm infants. Cochrane Database of Systematic Reviews. 2003;(2):CD000143

[24] Miller MJ, Carlo WA, Martin RJ. Continuous positive pressure selectively reduces obstructive apnea in preterm infants. Journal of Pediatrics. 1985;**106**:91-94

[25] Casey JL, Newberry D, Jnah A. Early bubble continuous positive airway pressure: Investigating interprofessional best practices for the NICU team. Neonatal Network. 2016;**35**(3):125-134

[26] Yagui ACZ, Vale LAPA, Haddad LB, Prado C, Rossi FS, Agostini Deutsch AD, et al. Bubble CPAP versus CPAP with variable flow in newborns with respiratory distress: A randomized controlled trial. Jornal de Pediatria. 2011;**87**(6):499-450

[27] Liptsen E, Aghai ZH, Pyon KH, Saslow JG, Nakhla T, Long J, et al. Work of breathing during nasal continuous positive airway pressure in preterm infants: A comparison of bubble

vs variable flow devices. Journal of Perinatology. 2005;**25**:453-458

[28] Davis P, Davies M, Faber B. A randomised controlled trial of two methods of delivering nasal continuous positive airway pressure after extubation to infants weighing less than 1,000 g: Binasal (Hudson) versus single nasal prongs. Archives of Disease in Childhood. Fetal and Neonatal Edition. 2001;**85**(2):F82-F85

[29] Morley CJ, Davis PG, Doyle LW, Brion LP, Hascoet JM, Carlin JB, et al. Nasal CPAP or intubation at birth for very preterm infants. The New England Journal of Medicine. 2008;**358**(7):700-708

[30] Thukral A, Sankar MJ, Chandrasekaran A, Agarwal R, Paul VK. Efficacy and safety of CPAP in low- and middle-income countries. Journal of Perinatology. 2016;**36**:S21-S28

[31] Abdel-Latif SME, Davis PG, Wheeler KI, De Paoli AG, Dargavill PA. Surfactant therapy via thin catheter in preterm infants with or at risk of respiratory distress syndrome. Cochrane Database of Systematic Review. 10 May 2021;**5**(5):CD011672. DOI: 10.1002/14651858. CD011672.pub2

[32] American Association for Respiratory Care. Clinical practice guideline. Application of continuous positive airway pressure to neonates via nasal prongs, nasopharyngeal tube, or nasal mask—2004 revision and update. Respiratory Care. 2004;**49**(9):11

[33] De Paoli AG, Davis PG, Faber B, Morley CJ. Devices and pressure sources for administration of nasal continuous airways pressure (nCPAP) in preterm infants. The Cochrane Collaboration. Cochrane Database of Systematic Review. 23 Jan 2008;**2008**(1):CD002977. DOI: 10.1002/14651858.CD002977.pub2

[34] Harris H, Wilson S, Brans Y, Wirtschafter D, Cassady G. Nasal continuous positive airway pressure. Improvement in arterial oxygenation in hyaline membrane disease. Biology of the Neonate. 1976;**29**(3-4):231-237. DOI: 10.1159/000240868

[35] King BC, Gandhi BB, Jackson A, Katakam L, Pammi M, Suresh G. Mask versus prongs for nasal continuous positive airway pressure in preterm infants: A systematic review and meta-analysis. Neonatology. 2019;**116**:100-114

[36] Verder H, Robertson B, Griesen G, et al. The Danish-Swedish multicentre study group. Surfactant therapy and nasal continuous positive airway pressure for newborns with respiratory distress syndrome. New England Journal of Medicine. 1994;**331**:1051-1055

[37] Dargaville PA, Gerber A, Johansson S, De Paoli AG, Kamlin CO, Orsini F, et al. Australian and New Zealand Neonatal Network. Incidence and outcome of CPAP failure in preterm infants. Pediatrics. 2016;**138**(1):e20153985. DOI: 10.1542/peds.2015-3985

[38] Dargaville PA, Gerber A, Johansson S, De Paoli AG, Kamlin COF, Orsini F, et al. Incidence and outcome of CPAP failure in preterm infants. Pediatrics. 2016;**138**(1):e20153985. DOI: 10.1542/peds.2015-3985

[39] Pillai MS, Sankar MJ, Mani K, Agarwal R, Paul VK, Deorari AK. Clinical prediction score for nasal CPAP failure in pre-term VLBW neonates with early onset respiratory distress. Journal of Tropical Pediatrics. 2011;**57**(4):274-279. DOI: 10.1093/tropej/fmq047

[40] Kattwinkel J, Fleming D, Cha CC, Fanaroff AA, Klaus MH. A device for administration of continuous positive

airway pressure by the nasal route. Pediatrics. 1973;**52**:131-134

[41] Stevens TP, Blennow M, Myers EH, Soll R. Early surfactant administration with brief ventilation vs. selective surfactant and continued mechanical ventilation for preterm infants with or at risk for respiratory distress syndrome. Cochrane Database of Systematic Reviews. 17 Oct 2007;**2007**(4):CD003063. DOI: 10.1002/14651858.CD003063.pub3

[42] Soll R, Ozek E. Prophylactic protein free synthetic surfactant for preventing morbidity and mortality in preterm infants. Cochrane Database of Systematic Reviews. 20 Jan 2010;(1):CD001079. DOI: 10.1002/14651858.CD001079.pub2

[43] Ahluwalia JS, White DK, Morley CJ. Single prong CPAP, either nasopharyngeal or short nasal, is a relatively simple technique. Infant flow driver or single prong nasal continuous positive airway pressure: Short-term physiological effects. Acta Paediatrica. 1998;**87**:325-327

[44] Minocchieri S, Berry CA, Pillow J. Nebulised surfactant to reduce severity of respiratory distress: A blinded, parallel, randomised controlled trial on behalf of the CureNeb Study Tea. Archives of Disease in Childhood. Fetal and Neonatal Edition. BMJ. May 2019;**104**(3):F313-F319. DOI: 10.1136/archdischild-2018-315051. [Epub 2018 Jul 26]

Chapter 7

# The Role of Leadership in Sub-Saharan Africa in Promoting Maternal and Child Health

*Zacharie Tsala Dimbuene, Tilahun Haregu, Raphaël Muanza Nzuzi and Paul-Denis Nzita Kikhela*

**Abstract**

Sub-Saharan Africa (SSA) continues to face adverse maternal and child health (MCH) outcomes compared to other regions of the world. Previous research showed that SSA countries did not reach Millennium Development Goals (MDG)-4 and MDG-5. To further our understanding of levels and correlates of MCH outcomes, numerous studies have focused on socioeconomic factors, both at individual, household, and community levels. This chapter adopted a different approach and emphasized the role of leadership at regional, national, and local levels to improve MCH outcomes in SSA countries. Overall, the chapter demonstrated that without an enlightened leadership, SSA countries will be lagging behind SDG-3 targets. Additionally, evidence to guide policymaking in most countries is lacking mainly due to lack of sound data to specifically meet the needs of policymakers. There is an urgent need to focus on Research and Development (R&D) and Innovation. To achieve this goal, a crucial shift in leadership is compulsory.

**Keywords:** leadership, governance and public policy, maternal and child health, universal health coverage, Sustainable Development Goals, sub-saharan Africa

## 1. Introduction

This chapter draws from the international agendas, Millennium Development Goals (MDGs) for 2000–2015 and the Sustainable Development Goals (SDGs) for 2015–2030 to highlight the role of leadership in promoting maternal and child health (hereafter, MCH) in sub-Saharan Africa (SSA). These perspectives set out to ensure acceptable levels of MCH outcomes across regions and countries, and within countries. For instance, under MDGs, the international agenda aims at reducing child mortality (MDG-4) and improve maternal health (MDG-5) [1]. However, only six countries (Botswana, Cape Verde, Eritrea, Malawi, Mauritius, and Seychelles) were on track to achieve Millennium Development Goal (MDG)-4, to reduce under-five mortality rate (U5MR) by two-thirds by 2015 [2]. Similarly, evidence showed many SSA countries were making insufficient progress in achieving MDG-5 of reducing the maternal mortality ratio (MMR) by three-quarters by 2015 [3]. It is therefore not surprising that research about maternal, newborn, and child health (MNCH) remains a top priority in the post-2015 development agenda. The new development agenda specifically sets out in goal 3 to “ensure healthy lives and promote well-being for all at all ages” including reducing MMR to 70 per 100,000 live births and neonatal mortality to as low as 12 per 1000 live births and under-five mortality to as low as 25 per 1000 live births. Worldwide, SSA countries are the greatest contributors of most preventable maternal and child deaths [4], yet an improvement of MCH in this region could lead to substantial reduction of maternal and child morbidity and mortality. In sum, most SSA countries did not reach MDG-4 and MDG-5, and likely they will not reach SDG-3. Therefore, this chapter answers the following overarching question: “Why SSA countries might not achieve SDG-3?” It posits that envisioned leadership, which is of paramount importance to achieving this goal, is crucially lacking in the region.

## 2. Sub-Sharan Africa: the world of poverty and hunger

In the past decade, the world has experienced significant socioeconomic progress, even though the effects of the COVID-19 pandemic have had negative effects on population wellbeing [5]. In this chapter, the Human Development Index (HDI) is used to show the inequalities across world regions and within region, essentially SSA. The underlying assumption is that poverty and hunger are rampant in countries with low HDI. Furthermore, it is unlike to expect sustainable health, including MCH, if people are not fed properly, and live in extreme poverty. The recent report on HDI shows the following. First, SSA is the least developed region in the world based on HDI. Indeed, HDI in developing regions range from 0.547 in SSA to 0.705 in Arab states. It is clear that the region is still facing a number of challenges, including leadership and governance, women’s empowerment, education, and employment among others. Turning to the distribution of HDI at country level, the report clearly shows that most SSA countries are located at the bottom of the ranking. For instance, 31 SSA countries ranked between 157th (Mauritania) and 187th position (Niger). This is a clear indication of poor leadership and governance in the region, adding up armed conflict and wars which are literally impeding sustainable democracies in the countries. Furthermore, the AIDS pandemic is still causing a number of serious damages in SSA countries, leaving behind vulnerable children and increasing the percentage of populations living under the poverty line [6]. Additionally, policymakers paid less attention to nutrition, while SSA is the region of the world where the number of underweight children has stagnated over time as a clear alarm to detrimental effects of malnutrition on children development growth, with all known consequences such as brain development [7–9]. Yet, fully complete nutrition is key to ensure optimal development and to ensure citizens are prepared to build national wealth while fighting hunger and eliminating poverty.

There is evidence of the co-occurrence of poverty and hunger in many regions of the world, including SSA and scholars really wonder if extreme poverty in SSA can be eliminated by 2030 [10, 11]. According to the World Bank, households with a per capita income or expenditure less than $1.90 per person per day are defined being poor [12]. From the Economic Development Report released recently [13], there is evidence that most SSA countries have made progress in reducing the number of people living below the poverty line. In fact, between 2010 and 2019, the percentage of households living below the poverty line ($1.9 per person per day) declined from 40 to 34%, in spite of the COVID-19 pandemic. It is common that people living in poverty to be undernourished, which led scholars to question the relationship between poverty and nutrition by adopting the human capital approach: Is it the cause or the consequence? Scholars posit that nutritional status has a profound impact on human capital [14], especially at earlier ages where the brain continues to develop. In the search of pathways of influence, scholars posited that malnutrition has adverse consequences on physical and mental health/development, productivity, and the economic potential of an individual. Likewise, poverty and malnutrition both affect MCH in the following ways. Poverty can be a strong barrier to access good healthcare services on the one hand [15–17], and on the other hand, malnutrition can be detrimental for maternal and child health [18].

Although most SSA countries made progress to reduce poverty levels amid the COVD-19 pandemic, the region is still lagging very behind compared with other regions in the world. Therefore, it is important to further our understanding of structural barriers impeding most SSA countries from meeting SDGs targets on maternal and child health. Before moving there, let us take a look on common indicators of MCH in the region.

## 3. Maternal and child health in sub-Saharan Africa: key indicators

This section addresses a number of MCH in sub-Saharan Africa, including antenatal care services, skilled birth attendant, facility-based delivery, utilization of postnatal care services, child health services, HIV testing, and prevention of mother-child transmission.

### 3.1 Antenatal care service coverage

Indicators to monitoring antenatal care services include, among others, utilization, frequency, and timing of ANC [17]. This chapter reports on two ANC indicators: (*i*) percentage of women who received four or more ANC visits during pregnancy according to WHO recommendations [19] and (*ii*) percentage of women who received ANC visit from a skilled provider (**Figure 1**). The number of women of reproductive ages in SSA countries has increased over time [20]. Data were available for 32 countries and findings showed that, on average, 56% of women received at least four visits during pregnancy. This figure ranged from 29.2% in Senegal to 90.5% in Ghana. Likely, Ghana has made tremendous progress in ANC coverage and access mainly due to a developed national insurance scheme [21] The percentage of women of reproductive ages who received antenatal care from a skilled provider was even higher on average in 36 countries with available data. Indeed, 88% of women received ANC visits from a skilled provided. While SSA countries made incredible progress on this area, there still are significant differences across countries. The lowest (51.6%) and highest (99.2%) percentages were observed in Togo and Burundi, respectively. It is worthy to mention that these two countries are among smallest countries in SSA in terms of superficies which can be a key element allowing national governments to better serve women of reproductive ages during pregnancies, a major cause of maternal deaths in the region.

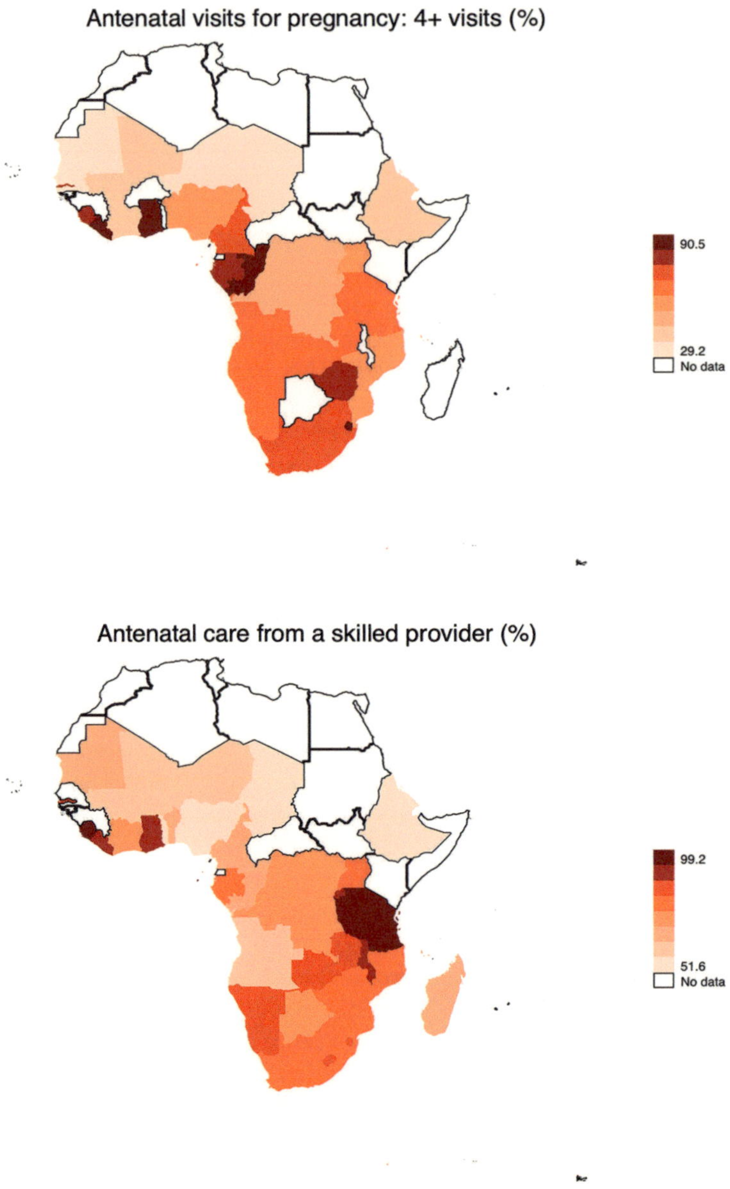


**Figure 1.**
*Antenatal care utilization in sub-Saharan Africa.*

Sub-Saharan Africa has a long history of Knowledge-Attitudes-Practices (KAP) studies since 1980s to better understand knowledge, attitudes, and practices of modern contraction among women of reproductive ages. It was expected like it was in the case of Asian Tigers that after more than four decades women have embraced modern contraception as a path to reduce/control the persistent higher fertility levels in the region. The reality is that women of reproductive ages in the region are still suffering of unmet needs for family planning (**Figure A.1**, appendix). Yet, without universal access to family planning, the population will continue to grow, even faster.

*DOI: http://dx.doi.org/10.5772/intechopen.105773*

### 3.2 Skilled birth attendance

Skilled birth attendance (SBA) has attracted much attention three decades ago when the Safe Motherhood campaign was launched in Kenya [22, 23]. It is posited that SBA can substantially reduce maternal deaths when skilled birth attendants (e.g. doctors) assist women during deliveries [22, 24–27]. Therefore, many preventable deaths during pregnancies in SSA are due to the quality of health professionals who assist women during deliveries. Data available on 28 countries indicated that, on average, 71% of women were assisted by a skilled professional at delivery, which contrasts a bit with the alarming level of maternal deaths in the region (**Figure 2**). Perhaps, the inequalities across countries concerning access to a skilled provided may explain the higher number of maternal deaths which is observed in the region. Indeed, only one-fourth of women of reproductive ages are assisted by a skilled birth attendant, while the corresponding figure is 96.7% in South Africa [25]. There are two things worthy to point out here. First, reliable data to provide evidence on the state of skilled birth attendance are still missing. Governments in SSA countries and the AU council should engage in providing sufficient finding to collect data supporting planning, implementation, and monitoring of MCH programs in the region at national and subnational levels. Second, it seems there is a correlation between the level of socioeconomic development and access to SBA when one looks into the bottom (Chad) and the top (South Africa). Further research could devote much attention on this hypothesis and if confirmed, this means that collective efforts in the region should be done to reduce these inequalities across countries.

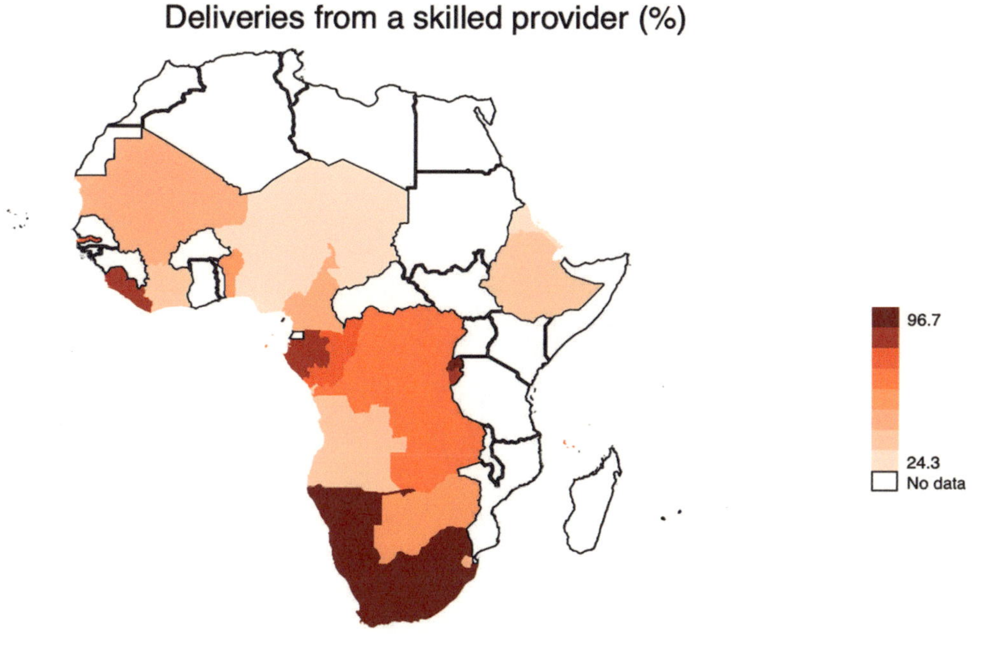


**Figure 2.**
*Skilled birth attendance in sub-Saharan Africa.*

### 3.3 Under-five mortality

Under-five mortality rate (U5MR), referred to as the probability to die before the fifth anniversary, is a key indicator to measure the socio-development of a country and child health [28–30]. In the last few decades, tremendous progress has been done to reduce the probability of a live birth to die before his/her fifth birthday, even though the levels of U5MR still are higher in SSA countries compared with other regions in the world. Yet, it is important to identify appropriate targets and devise effective interventions if SSA countries to reduce mortality among children under 5 years of age [28]. Again, that is where leadership comes into play because main causes of infant morbidity and mortality have been extensively studied worldwide and the region, but still progress has been very limited so for. Data from 29 countries showed that SSA countries register on average 83 deaths per 1000 live births (**Figure 3**). Alarmingly, this figure is far above the target of SDG-3.2 which aims 25 deaths per 1000 live births [31]. Furthermore, there are significant inequalities across SSA countries which need to be tackled collectively if national Governments want to reach SDG-3.2 [32]. Indeed, U5MR ranged from 41 deaths per 1000 live births in Mauritania to 158 deaths per 1000 live births in Central African Republic. Additional efforts targeting Central Africa are crucial to improve child health as shown in this chapter. A previous work showed that socioeconomic indicators are worse in Central Africa compared with other regions in the region [33]. The region has also been

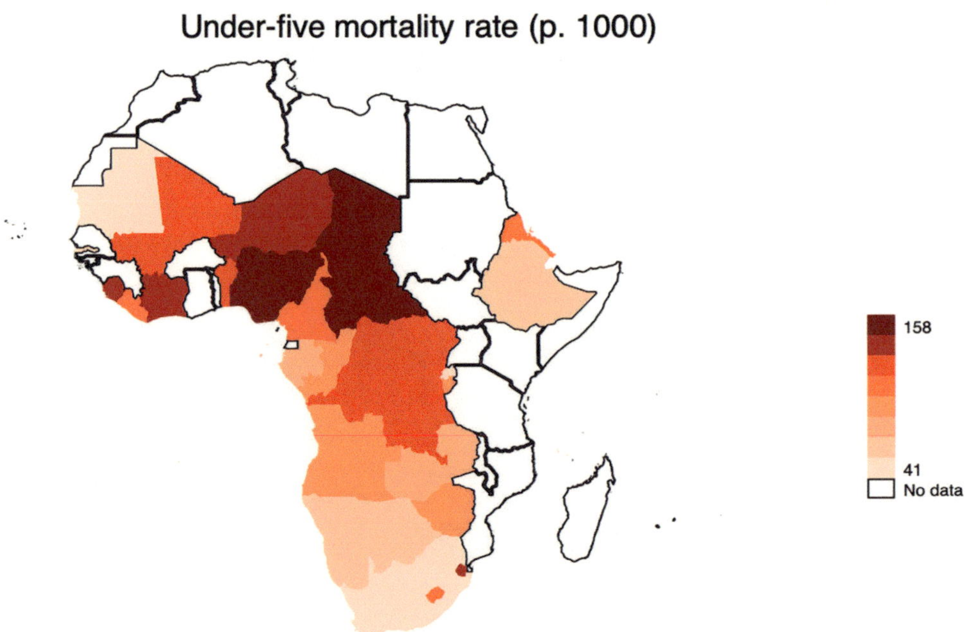


**Figure 3.**
*Under-five mortality rate in sub-Saharan Africa.*

suffering with poor leadership through dictatorship and armed conflict. For instance, the Democratic Republic of the Congo has suffered since 1965 with poor leadership, lack of transparency, corruption, among others. Likewise, Central African Republic has been very unstable and until now, the country does not have effective government due to armed conflict. Gabon, the Republic of Congo, and Cameroon have been relatively stable, but they lack clear vision and accountability, and rampant corruption is knocking the doors every time. Such context is not conducive to boost economic development, and thereafter, improve MCH in the countries.

### 3.4 Child health: stunting and wasting

Over the last four decades, child (mal)nutrition has crystalized interest in both scientific and policymaking spheres [34–37] for several reasons. First, child malnutrition is a major public concern in SSA countries; it represents both a cause and a manifestation of poverty. Second, poor nutrition among young children has short- and long-term consequences. For instance, child malnutrition increases the risks of morbidity from infectious diseases and mortality; it affects cognitive and mental/brain development and work productivity in adulthood. Finally, there is increasingly evidence that poor nutrition yields to poor reproductive outcomes, obesity, and chronic diseases in later life [7, 9, 34, 38–42]. At some point, one might wonder if poor brain development could explain the rampant poor leadership observed in SSA countries. First, most "leaders" come from poor households where they suffered from poor nutrition in their 1000 first days in life. Second, most people ruling did not have a chance to attend kindergarten where children are taught good behaviors in early life, such as sharing, listening, respect, love, among others. Turning back to data available on 27 countries (**Figure 4**), findings indicated that on average, 32% of children are stunted, with significant geographical variations in the region. Indeed, the percentage of children stunted varies from 16.5% in Gabon to 55.9% in Burundi. Such figures do not health in achieving SDG-3.2, since poor nutritional status among children is a major cause of morbidity and mortality. Furthermore, previous studies have documented the interlinkages between slow growth in height during childhood and impaired health, and poor school and economic performance [8, 9, 43]. With regard to wasting, findings showed that on average, 6.6% of children are affected. The lowest and highest percentage of wasted children were observed in Rwanda (1.1%) and Niger (18.0%), respectively. Like stunting, wasting during gestation and childhood has short- and long-term consequences later in life [44]. The Dutch famine of 1944 –1945 is illustrative of such chaos [45]. This study showed that exposure to famine during gestation resulted in antisocial personality and affective disorders, among others. Yet, these traits are very important to develop/foster a strong leadership. Even though people ruling developed countries are not perfect, one might admit that commitments toward public service are likely indication of social personality and affective traits, which in turn engage rulers to build their countries and treat people well somehow. In contrast, people ruling SSA countries do not feel accountable, more likely because they have antisocial personality and affective disorders, as a result of poor nutrition during pregnancy and early childhood.

Within this background showing clearly that key indicators of MCH are SSA countries is still of great concern while being a major public health issue, the region needs a significant shift through a strategic vision and leadership to devise and implement sound policies to improve MCH and therefore help SSA countries to achieve globally SDG-3.

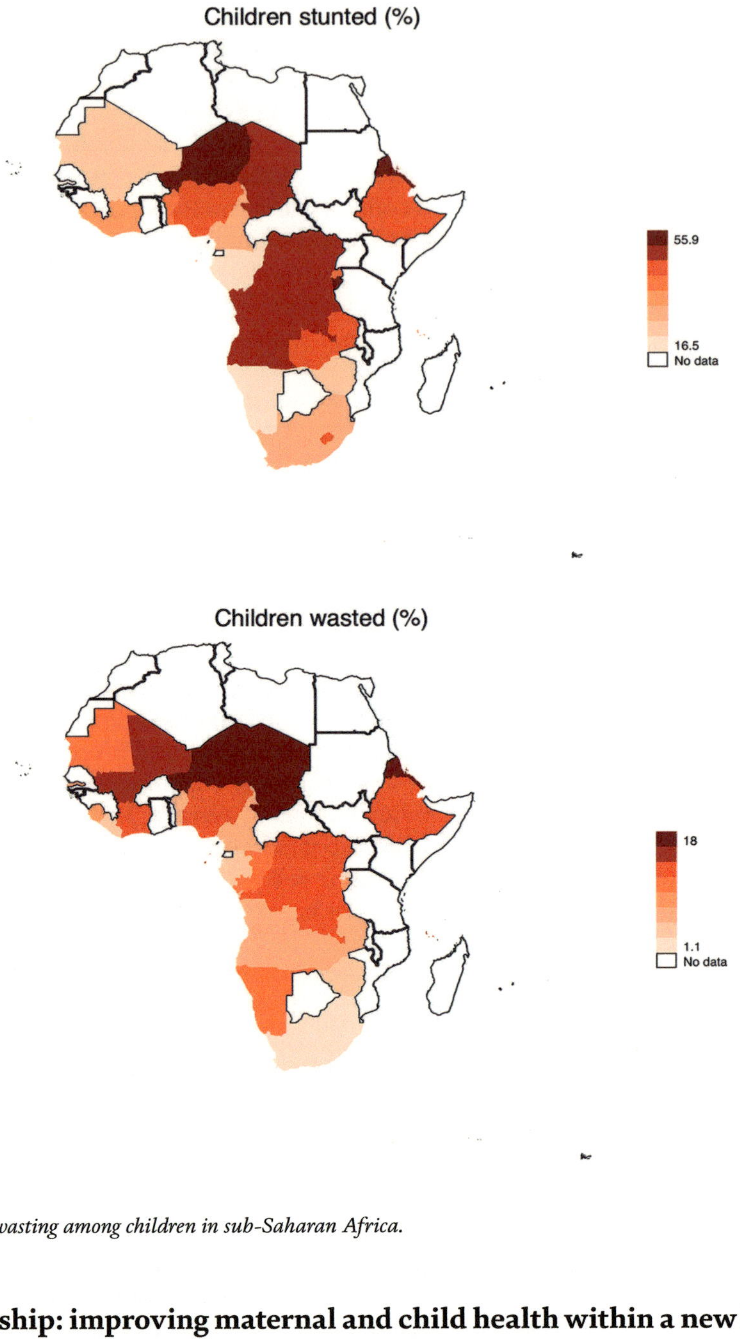


**Figure 4.**
*Stunting and wasting among children in sub-Saharan Africa.*

## 4. Leadership: improving maternal and child health within a new lens

As aforementioned, SSA is one of the poorest regions on the earth in spite of plenty resources in the SSA countries. That is where leadership comes into play as it is usually posited that "to great evils, great remedies." In this chapter, it is assumed that a transformational leadership is compulsory for SSA countries to achieve SDGs and substantially improve MCH in the region in the context of weak economies and heightened pressures for action, including global economic crisis and austerity politics, demographic changes [46], and increasing inequity of maternal healthcare utilization between poor and rich [17], and amid the rampant consequences of urban poverty [16], and the unstoppable effects of COVID-19 in SSA.

Kuhlmann et al. offer an interesting perspective to further our understanding of healthcare policy and governance within an integrative approach to include, among others, policies and governance to ensure universal coverage, access to healthcare, financing, quality of care, and health equity [46]. Deepening all these areas is beyond the scope of this chapter. These notions have been extensively discussed elsewhere [47]. Furthermore, previous research clearly identified eight governance principles to account for to better activate the workplace in health sector [48]. These include information, accountability, strategic vision, transparency, efficiency, equity, responsiveness, and voice and participation. More importantly, they pointed out to leadership as a key action in Health Action Framework. Turning now on what should be the role of leadership in enhancing MCH in sub-Saharan Africa, this chapter borrows from the demographic dividend (DD) to sharpen its importance in the MCH context (see **Figure 5**).

The overarching question from **Figure 5** stems from the precedence in the "enabling environment" to more likely reach the goal of improved maternal and child health in sub-Saharan Africa, while assuming all factors (education, health, economics, and governance) are important. In a previous work, I argued that governance was the most important piece to manage if SSA countries wanted successfully to reach SDGs, and specifically SDG-3. Before expanding on the role of leadership on MCH in SSA, let us revisit what scholars have done so far regarding the role of governance on MCH.

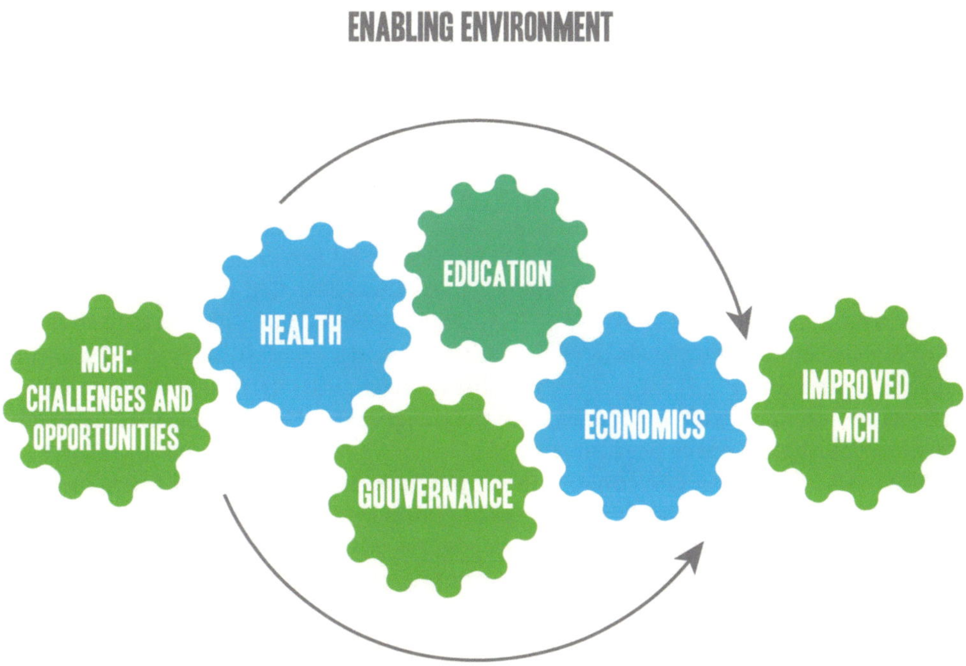


**Figure 5.**
*Pathways to improved maternal and child outcomes in sub-Saharan Africa.*

### 4.1 Governance and maternal and child health in sub-Saharan Africa

There are several attempts to address the importance of governance in SSA concerning challenges and opportunities to substantially improve MCH at both national, subnational, and local levels [18, 49–52]. These studies identified strengths and weaknesses. Kaplan et al. provide a good summary of strengths and weaknesses within the human resource perspective [48]. Strengths include among others, increasing transparency of financial flows and responsiveness to population needs through training of new cadres of health workers to address shortages and deliver care to more vulnerable populations and remote areas; implementing pilot programs that apply financial and nonfinancial incentives which ultimately increase efficiency; and easing onboarding process for health workers. Regarding weaknesses, most countries lack to develop, implement, and evaluate health workforce policies that outline a strategic vision, to implement accountability regulations in the health workforce, and to use health information systems to provide evidence for better decision-making. However, as shown later, most interventions to strengthening governance in healthcare have mainly focused on the use of resources. Indeed, Schneider et al. showed that initiatives to strengthen the governance of district health systems in South Africa which are pivotal to reach SDG-3 have used various methodologies [52], and therefore results are not necessarily comparable on the one hand, and on the other hand, have focused on improving the efficiency of resource use. This is likely because most SSA countries spend less moment in national budgets and mostly rely on public aid on development (PAD), with high control over resource is a requirement to benefit PAD. But overall, governance in SSA countries has been ineffective given the results obtained in terms of improving MCH in these countries. There is still then an unanswered question, why is governance so ineffective in SSA countries yet it is of crucial importance to boost MCH in this deprived region of world? This chapter addresses this question in the next section.

### 4.2 Leadership and maternal and child health in sub-Saharan Africa

The interlinkages between governance and leadership are important to catch up at a glance if one might understand the chief importance of leadership in shaping MCH in SSA countries. There are many reasons to seriously address the role of leadership in the context of MCH in SSA. First, and as it was shown earlier, the region is lagging very behind in terms of socioeconomic indicators. Second, the region is the most politically unstable region in the world. The recent coups in Mali, Burkina Faso, and Guinea may tell us more. Third, there are almost no indications that the region will perform well in the next few decades with the observable effects of COVID-19 placing SSA in the most vulnerable position [53, 54].

What is governance? The concept is not new and has been over decades in political and academic spheres. Governance comprises collective actions and measures adopted by a group of people to achieve common goals [55]. According to The World Bank, collective actions and measures are not an end, instead they should be guided by a number of formal and unformal rules [56]. According to Rhodes, "governance refers to: a new process of governing; or a changed condition of ordered rule; or the new method by which society is governed" [57]. In practice and for the best of people's wellbeing, the international community has introduced the concept of "good governance" as opposed to "poor governance" which is a multifaceted concept comprising eight factors, including Participation, Rule of

Law, Transparency, Responsiveness, Consensus Oriented, Equity and Inclusiveness, Effectiveness and Efficiency, and Accountability [58]. All these components are important; however, responsiveness refers to as the leadership required to boost the collective actions and measures taken by the national governments. Therefore, one might question the interlinkages between leadership and effective MCH interventions in SSA countries.

This chapter builds on a modified framework from policy interventions facilitating demographic dividend (see **Figure 5**) [59]. There have been several attempts to address the linkages between leadership and MCH; however, they have mainly focused on "lower levels" targeting professionals and cadres in health workforce [60–64]. Most studies have focused on capacity-building, development of skills to better serve more deprived segments of the population, and accountability. Although this research agenda is quite important, this chapter posits that it is not sufficient to reach SDG-3 given the results obtained during the MDG momentum. Therefore, it is of paramount importance to bring the debate at higher levels to expect a substantial shift which can really change the current situation of MCH in SSA, including the African Union (AU)'s and country's commitments to improve MCH in the region. This is not unexpectable because countries such as Thailand or Korea have shown such great successes in the past to improve population wellbeing, including maternal and child health [15, 65, 66].

#### *4.2.1 Maternal and child health in sub-Saharan Africa: AU agenda*

In 2016, the African Union (AU) discussed its heath strategy in Addis Ababa in preparation of the 2016 meeting of Ministers of Health in Geneva, Switzerland, in May 2016 [67]. In the situation analysis, one might read that the "region still faces urgent need to accelerate progress" toward (*i*) improving child health. Indeed, even though a decline of 40% in infant mortality rate (IMR) between 1990 and 2014 from 90 deaths per 1000 live births to 54 deaths per 1000 live births, there still are substantial variations across and within countries, and therefore impeding the regions to reach SDG-3. Furthermore, the region still experiences a significant percentage of unmet need for modern contraceptives estimated at 26% which has almost flattened between 1990 and 2013.

Expectedly, the AU report pointed out the path to better MCH outcomes as it indicated that top-level commitment, stewardship, accountability, and transparency in the leadership and governance within the health sector are critical to improve health in SSA countries in general, and specifically MCH. It also extended saying that SSA countries should consider instituting effective decentralization of functions, authority, and resources to improve health sector performance. However, the report is silent about the time horizon on the one hand, and on the other hand it does not provide any indication of dictatorship and centralized power in the region, and how they are detrimental to achieve good health [68]. Previous research showed that despite of some progress made in SSA countries to improve maternal healthcare utilization [17], there are increasing inequalities between poor and rich and this might impede the progress observed so far.

The report mentioned among other strategic approaches, health research, and innovation as a transformational path to health sector and the African economy as a whole by suggesting an investment of 2% of the national budget in Science and Technology between 2014 and 2024. The reality is that Research & Development still unfunded (or at least poorly funded) in most SSA countries. Most initiatives of research funding are foreign/international, and therefore, they do not sound and sustainable research on the one hand, and on the other hand, they might overlook specific needs of SSA countries. For instance, the Innovating for Maternal and Child Health in Africa (IMCHA) Initiative aimed at improving maternal and child health in SSA countries through research and was funded by International Development Research Centre (IRDC) of Canada [69]. The project is certainly worthy since it addresses critical knowledge gaps and increases awareness among policymakers; however, it is not sufficient to provoke a significant shift in the organization of health systems in most SSA countries without enlightened leadership from national and local governments in SSA countries. First, the project was geographically unbalanced since it was led in 11 countries. Second, the project less focused on ownership of the outcomes, and it is not obvious that policymakers will use the generated knowledge to implement sound policies to improve MCH in SSA countries. Likewise, African Population and Health Research Center (APHRC) in Nairobi (Kenya), the 2015 UNFPA Population Award, has been doing since 2000s such an incredible job in generating knowledge and evidence for the African continent [70]. This organization operates through international research grants since its inception and has rarely benefited money from African governments to undertake research which African-funded, African-led research, and context-specific. Observers would ask themselves if African governments do really understand the importance of research and evidence-based policymaking. It is time to make the shift if SSA countries want to achieve SDG-3.

#### *4.2.2 Maternal and child health in sub-Saharan Africa: country-level commitments and progress*

The last section focused on the highest level of commitment, the AU agenda. The most functional level, the country level, is pivotal in implementing sound programs and policies to expect progress in MCH indicators. The section expands on the previous one and borrows main ideas from **Figure 5**. The enabling environment is critical for a country to achieve optimal maternal and child health, while significantly reducing the poor-rich inequality and eliminating urban advantage. But in this search of the "quality of MCH," what is the best enabling mechanism? Of course, education, health, economics, and governance are all important. However, to optimize the achievement of universal health coverage within the lens of MCH, national governments should decide where or what to focus on first and foremost. What need to be done to efficiently utilize resources to create good quality of MCH services? How long did it take to reach SDG-3?

These questions are complementary but even more complex. For instance, what will be the added value in terms of MCH outcomes when healthcare workforce is well trained but not well paid? Just take a minute and think about the Arab spring and all consequences of the long-term frustration in the region, which have devastated the fragile economies. There is an urgent need to critically think of the best way to articulate education and motivation in the health sector in SSA countries. Relatedly, what will happen if human resources are well trained but are employed in small jobs that do not fit their skills? It is a human being instinct to survive. If a well-trained health professional cannot find a job that really fits his/her skills, he/she will take whichever given job to survive. This impeding situation will lead to demotivation and less productivity as the individual will always be thinking of another work and will not be creative as he/she would have been in a job-matching context. In this case, education has a less added value than in a conducive environment.

The paper posits that what happened in "Asian Tigers" to put their economies in right paths and implement sound policies that improved population wellbeing and health is a "manifestation of enlightened and strong leadership," which was able to guide public opinions and behaviors. In 2015, African Union for Population Studies (UAPS) organized its 7th Population Conference in Pretoria (South Africa) under the theme "Demographic dividend in Africa: Prospects, opportunities, and challenges" which registered a high number of papers and presentations, and interesting debate about how sub-Saharan Africa can reap demographic dividend. Dr. Prata presented a paper entitled "Access to family planning and women's health." Using a graph from a previous study to illustrate the relationship between fertility, contraception, and abortion in Korea between 1960 and 2000 [71], Dr. Prata pointed out a striking fact in her presentation to highlight the major differences between SSA countries and the Asian Tigers. The Korean experience showed that the initial stage of fertility decline was accompanied by both increases in contraception and abortion for more than 15 years. However, the difference between SSA and Korea was that Korean women had access to safe abortion, while SSA still experience unsafe and high abortion rates. This illustration symbolizes how policy decisions may have greater impact than simple vows.

Back to our question about the gradient among the enablers and put differently, while the world is vibrating at the rhythm of SDGs and demographic dividend, the paper assumes that "Governance" should be the most important pillar to drive the necessary and sufficient decisions for SSA countries to reach SDG-3. Let us use malaria as a simple case for illustration. It is well known that malaria still is one of the major causes of death in SSA account for 94% of deaths [72], and it is also well known that SSA countries have poorest MCH indicators worldwide. This endemic illness costs to Africa, the poorest continent of the planet, an amount of $US 12 billion in lost productivity and health expenditures per year [71]. It means that if SSA countries have worked together to find sustainable ways to fight malaria, they could have been able to save up to $US 12 billion to invest in other productive sectors to boost their economies and improve MCH outcomes. Likewise, better housing and investments in clean environments can mitigate the reproduction of mosquitoes in rural and urban areas and could have saved lives and money.

Both scientists and policymakers however are hiding behind the broad theme of "enabling environment" and unable to decode the black box "Enabling Environment." The terms "governance" seems vague and confusing in some sense, and it has become a condition for international aid. As seen rhetorically, it means "democracy" or "change of regime." Many SSA countries have witnessed changes of regime in the last decade; however, does it really mean "governance" or "good governance"? Admittedly, democracy and change of regime are ingredient to governance, but a transformational leadership capable to guide the countries in the right direction and responsibly address the bottlenecks impeding economic growth to improve population wellbeing is blatantly lacking in the region. SSA has experienced an average growth rate on gross domestic product (GDP); yet most of SSA countries have the lowest Human Development Index (HDI). That is what makes the difference between the Asian Tigers and SSA countries. Strong and transformational leadership in Asian Tigers had a vision and took the necessary policies to change their business models and boost economic growth. In SSA, it is intriguing that countries do not learn from past experiences: slavery, structural adjustment programs, democratization, political instability, and so on. All those factors are key to understand SSA's history and should guide our vision for the future. The same recipes will always produce to some extent the same results. SSA countries experienced very bad results worldwide on MDGs; they will likely experience the worst results for SDGs. Therefore, SDG-3 will be a futile slogan if there is no radical political shift of leadership in SSA countries. The problem is well known: SSA is suffering from a very poor leadership without a vision of what the governments want for their countries to stand for in the next few decades. SSA countries are comparable to machines without captains. Are we going to expect miracles without a clear roadmap? Absolutely not! Therefore, it is important for SSA governments to stop and see what they are doing well, and mostly what does not help their nations. SSA countries have the potential to reap demographic dividend; however, that should be accompanied by a shift in political will leading to a strong leadership and decisions benefiting the countries.

## 5. Conclusion: takeaway messages about leadership and MCH in SSA countries

This chapter has stressed the well-known socioeconomic disadvantage sub-Saharan Africa (SSA) is facing adverse maternal and child health (MCH) outcomes compared to other regions of the world. Essentially, it showed that most SSA countries did not reach Millennium Development Goals (MDG)-4 and MDG-5. Also, it is very likely that SSA countries will not achieve Sustainable Development Goals (SDG)-3 based on the actual progress of most countries in the region. Given the alarming landscape of the region regarding MCH, and based on previous work, the chapter has demonstrated that leadership plays a pivotal to boost MCH outcomes in the region on the one hand and to accelerate the socioeconomic development of the region as a whole. Indeed, most SSA countries have committed in international agenda about maternal and child health, and they all have policies and programs targeting MCH outcomes. However, significant progress toward targets on SDG-3 is rare in most countries. First, data are lacking to provide them with clear evidence to devise specific programs and interventions. On this matter, data revolution in the region is compulsory. Most sources of data, mainly Demographic and Health Surveys (DHS) and Multiple Indicators Surveys (MIS) are not funded by national/local governments. Therefore, there is a lack of ownership in the region and SSA countries. Second, research funding is lacking in most SSA countries; yet it is harder to think of development with Research and Development (R&D) and Innovation. Third, the region is struggling to get enlightened leaders with a clear vision to determine where their respective countries and the region is heading in the next 10 or 20 years.

## Acknowledgements

This research does not have any funding.

## Conflict of interest

The authors declare no conflict of interest.

## A. Appendix

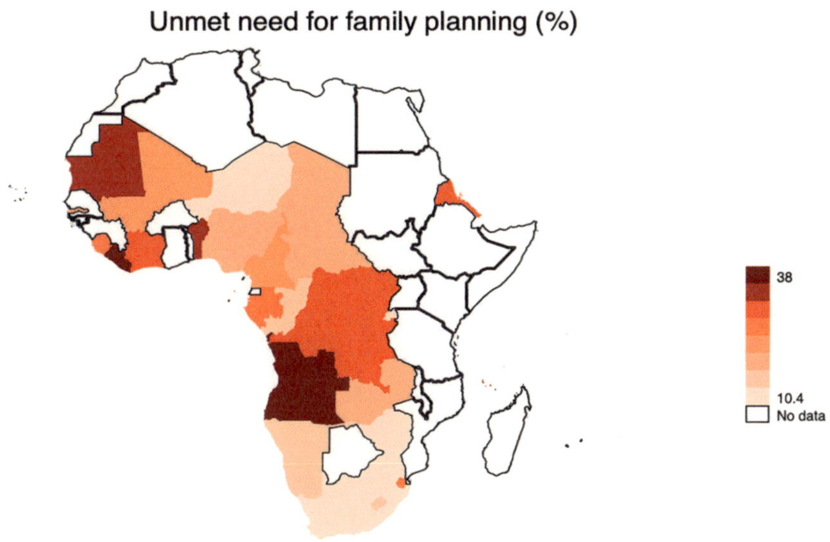


**Figure A.1.**
*Unmet needs for family planning in sub-Saharan Africa.*

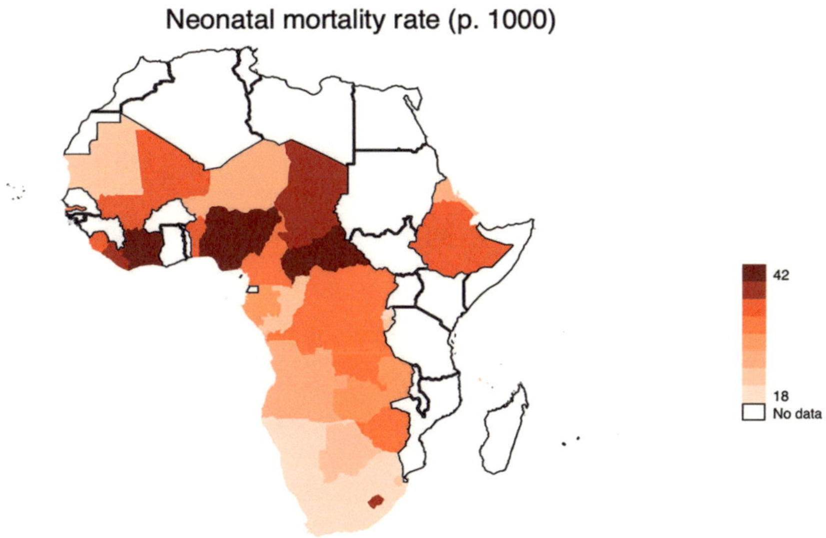


**Figure A.2.**
*Neonatal mortality rate in sub-Saharan Africa.*

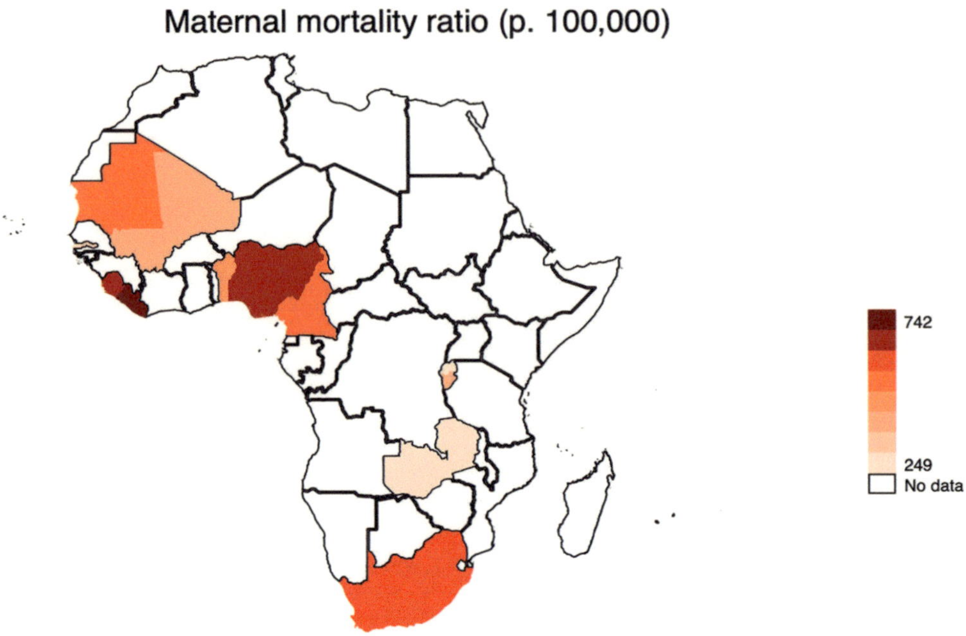


**Figure A.3.**
*Maternal mortality rate in sub-Saharan Africa.*

## Author details

Zacharie Tsala Dimbuene[1*], Tilahun Haregu[2], Raphaël Muanza Nzuzi[1] and Paul-Denis Nzita Kikhela[1]

1 Faculty of Economics and Management, Department of Population and Development Sciences, University of Kinshasa, Democratic Republic of the Congo

2 Nossal Institute for Global Health, University of Melbourne, Australia

*Address all correspondence to: zacharie.tsala.dimbuene@gmail.com

## References

[1] Haines A, Cassels A. Can the millennium development goals be attained? BMJ. 2004;**329**(7462):394-397

[2] Friberg IK, Kinney MV, Lawn JE, Kerber KJ, Odubanjo MO, Bergh AM, et al. Sub-saharan Africa's mothers, newborns, and children: How many lives could be saved with targeted health interventions? PLoS Medicine. 2010;7(6):e1000295

[3] Hogan MC, Foreman KJ, Naghavi M, Ahn SY, Wang M, Makela SM, et al. Maternal mortality for 181 countries, 1980-2008: A systematic analysis of progress towards Millennium Development Goal 5. The Lancet. 2010;**375**(9726):1609-1623

[4] Merdad L, Ali MM. Timing of maternal death: Levels, trends, and ecological correlates using sibling data from 34 sub-Saharan African countries. PLoS One. 2018;**13**(1):e0189416

[5] UNDP, editor. The Next Frontier: Human Development and the Anthropocene. United Nations Development Programme: New York, NY; 2020. p. 396

[6] Chopra M, Darnton-Hill I. Responding to the crisis in sub-Saharan Africa: The role of nutrition. Public Health Nutrition. 2006;**9**(5):544-550

[7] Cusick SE, Georgieff MK. The role of nutrition in brain development: The golden opportunity of the "First 1000 Days.". The Journal of Pediatrics. 2016;**175**:16-21

[8] Georgieff MK, Brunette KE, Tran PV. Early life nutrition and neural plasticity. Development and Psychopathology. 2015;**27**(2):411-423

[9] Prado EL, Dewey KG. Nutrition and brain development in early life. Nutrition Reviews. 2014;**72**(4):267-284

[10] Bicaba Z, Brixiová Z, Ncube M. Can Extreme Poverty in Sub-Saharan Africa be Eliminated by 2030? J Afr Dev. 2017;**19**(2):93-110

[11] Siddiqui F, Salam RA, Lassi ZS, Das JK. The intertwined relationship between malnutrition and poverty. Frontiers in Public Health. 2020;**8**. DOI: 10.3389/fpubh.2020.00453

[12] Heltberg R. Malnutrition, poverty, and economic growth. Health Economics. 2009;**18**(S1):S77-S88

[13] UNCTAD. Economic Development in Africa: Reaping the Potential Benefits of the African Continental Free Trade Area for Inclusive Growth. Geneva: United Nations; 2021. p. 204 (Economic development in Africa report)

[14] Setboonsarng S. Child Malnutrition as a Poverty Indicator: An Evaluation in the Context of Different Development Interventions in Indonesia. ADBI Discussion Paper; 2005. Report No.: 21. Available from: https://www.econstor.eu/handle/10419/53441

[15] Limwattananon S, Tangcharoensathien V, Prakongsai P. Equity in maternal and child health in Thailand. Bulletin of the World Health Organization. 2010;**88**(6):420-427

[16] Prakash R, Kumar A. Urban poverty and utilization of maternal and child health care services in India. Journal of Biosocial Science. 2013;**45**(4):433-449

[17] Tsala Dimbuene Z, Amo-Adjei J, Amugsi D, Mumah J, Izugbara CO,

Beguy D. Women's education and utilization of maternal health services in Africa: A multi-country and socioeconomic status analysis. Journal of Biosocial Science. 2018;**50**(6):725-748

[18] Keats EC, Das JK, Salam RA, Lassi ZS, Imdad A, Black RE, et al. Effective interventions to address maternal and child malnutrition: An update of the evidence. The Lancet Child & Adolescent Health. 2021;5(5):367-384

[19] World Health Organization (WHO). WHO Recommendations on Maternal and Newborn Care for a Positive Postnatal Experience. Geneva, Switzerland: WHO; 2022. p. 242. Available from: https://www.who.int/publications/i/item/9789240045989

[20] Sidze EM, Wekesah FM, Kisia L, Abajobir A. Inequalities in access and utilization of maternal, newborn and child health services in sub-Saharan Africa: A special focus on urban settings. Maternal and Child Health Journal. 2021;**26**:250-279. DOI: 10.1007/s10995-022-03396-4

[21] Blanchet NJ, Fink G, Osei-Akoto I. The effect of Ghana's national health insurance scheme on health care utilisation. Ghana Medical Journal. 2012;**46**(2):76-84

[22] Dickson KS, Adde KS, Ameyaw EK. Women empowerment and skilled birth attendance in sub-Saharan Africa: A multi-country analysis. PLoS One. 2021;**16**(7):e0254281

[23] Sai FT. The safe motherhood initiative: A call for action. IPPF Medical Bulletin. 1987;**21**(3):1-2

[24] Ameyaw EK, Dickson KS. Skilled birth attendance in Sierra Leone, Niger, and mali: Analysis of demographic and health surveys. BMC Public Health. 2020;**20**(1):164

[25] Bobo FT, Asante A, Woldie M, Dawson A, Hayen A. Spatial patterns and inequalities in skilled birth attendance and caesarean delivery in sub-Saharan Africa. BMJ Global Health. 2021;**6**(10):e007074

[26] Tessema ZT, Tesema GA. Pooled prevalence and determinants of skilled birth attendant delivery in East Africa countries: A multilevel analysis of Demographic and Health Surveys. Italian Journal of Pediatrics. 2020;**46**(1):177

[27] Zuñiga JA, García A, Kyololo OM, Hamilton-Solum P, Kabimba A, Milimo B, et al. Increasing utilisation of skilled attendants at birth in sub-Saharan Africa: A systematic review of interventions. International Journal of Nursing Studies. 2021;**120**:103977

[28] Perin J, Mulick A, Yeung D, Villavicencio F, Lopez G, Strong KL, et al. Global, regional, and national causes of under-5 mortality in 2000-19: An updated systematic analysis with implications for the Sustainable Development Goals. The Lancet Child & Adolescent Health. 2022;**6**(2):106-115

[29] Tesfa D, Tiruneh SA, Azanaw MM, Gebremariam AD, Engdaw MT, Kefale B, et al. Time to death and its determinants among under-five children in Sub-Saharan Africa using the recent (2010-2018) demographic and health survey data: Country-based shared frailty analyses. BMC Pediatrics. 2021;**21**(1):515

[30] Van Malderen C, Amouzou A, Barros AJD, Masquelier B, Van Oyen H, Speybroeck N. Socioeconomic factors contributing to under-five mortality in sub-Saharan Africa: A decomposition analysis. BMC Public Health. 2019;**19**(1):760

[31] UN general assembly. Transforming our world: The 2030 Agenda for

Sustainable Development. The Internet 2016. Available from: https://sustainabledevelopment.un.org/post2015/transformingourworld

[32] Moyer CA, Waiswa P. In-country data will illuminate under-5 mortality disparities. The Lancet. 2021;**398**(10303):821-822

[33] Pongou R, Kuate Defo B, Tsala DZ. Excess male infant mortality: The gene-institution interactions. The American Economic Review. 2017;**107**(5):541-545

[34] Adair LS, Guilkey DK. Age-specific determinants of stunting in filipino children. The Journal of Nutrition. 1997;**127**(2):314-320

[35] Fotso JC, Kuate-Defo B. Measuring socioeconomic status in health research in developing countries: Should we be focusing on households, communities or both? Social Indicators Research. 2005;**72**(2):189-237

[36] Fotso JC, Kuate-Defo B. Socioeconomic inequalities in early childhood malnutrition and morbidity: Modification of the household-level effects by the community SES. Health & Place. 2005;**11**(3):205-225

[37] UNICEF. The State of the World's Children 1998. New York: Oxford University Press; 1998

[38] DeLong GR. Effects of nutrition on brain development in humans. The American Journal of Clinical Nutrition. 1993;**57**(2):286S-290S

[39] Gopalan S. Malnutrition: Causes, consequences, and solutions. Nutrition. 2000;**7-8**(16):556-558

[40] Guesry P. The role of nutrition in brain development. Preventive Medicine. 1998;**27**(2):189-194

[41] De OM, Frongillo EA, Blössner M. Is malnutrition declining? An analysis of changes in levels of child malnutrition since 1980. Bulletin of the World Health Organization. 2000;**78**:1222-1233

[42] Ricci JA, Becker S. Risk factors for wasting and stunting among children in Metro Cebu, Philippines. The American Journal of Clinical Nutrition. 1996;**63**(6):966-975

[43] Dewey KG, Begum K. Long-term consequences of stunting in early life. Maternal & Child Nutrition. 2011;**7**(s3):5-18

[44] Wells JC, Sawaya AL, Wibaek R, Mwangome M, Poullas MS, Yajnik CS, et al. The double burden of malnutrition: Aetiological pathways and consequences for health. The Lancet. 2020;**395**(10217):75-88

[45] Kyle UG, Pichard C. The dutch famine of 1944-1945: A pathophysiological model of long-term consequences of wasting disease. Current Opinion in Clinical Nutrition and Metabolic Care. 2006;**9**(4):388-394

[46] Kuhlmann E, Blank RH, Bourgeault IL, Wendt C. Healthcare Policy and Governance in International Perspective. In: Kuhlmann E, Blank RH, Bourgeault IL, Wendt C, editors. The Palgrave International Handbook of Healthcare Policy and Governance. New York, NY: Palgrave Macmillan; 2015. pp. 3-22

[47] Kuhlmann E, Blank RH, Bourgeault IL, Wendt C, editors. The Palgrave International Handbook of Healthcare Policy and Governance. London: Palgrave Macmillan UK; 2015. DOI: 10.1057/9781137384935

[48] Kaplan AD, Dominis S, Palen JG, Quain EE. Human resource governance:

What does governance mean for the health workforce in low- and middle-income countries? Human Resources for Health. 2013;**11**(1):6

[49] Chen H, Chai Y, Dong L, Niu W, Zhang P. Effectiveness and appropriateness of mhealth interventions for maternal and child health: Systematic review. JMIR mHealth and uHealth. 2018;**6**(1):e8998

[50] Esamai F, Nangami M, Tabu J, Mwangi A, Ayuku D, Were E. A system approach to improving maternal and child health care delivery in Kenya: Innovations at the community and primary care facilities (a protocol). Reproductive Health. 2017;**14**(1):105

[51] Liu Y, Yang W. Leadership and governance tools for village sustainable development in China. Sustainability. 2019;**11**(20):5553

[52] Schneider H, George A, Mukinda F, Tabana H. District governance and improved maternal, neonatal and child health in South Africa: Pathways of Change. Health System Reform. 2020;**6**(1):e1669943

[53] Abubakar I, Dalglish SL, Angell B, Sanuade O, Abimbola S, Adamu AL, et al. The Lancet Nigeria Commission: investing in health and the future of the nation. The Lancet. 2022;**399**(10330):1155-1200

[54] Ajayi AI, Akpan W. Maternal health care services utilisation in the context of 'Abiye' (safe motherhood) programme in Ondo State, Nigeria. BMC Public Health. 2020;**20**(1):362

[55] Caulfield T, Hort K. Governance and Stewardship in Mixed Health Systems in Low- and Middle- Income Countries. Melbourne: The Nossal Institute for Global Health, The University of Melbourne; 2012

[56] World Bank Group. World Development Report 2017: Governance and the Law. Washington, DC: World Bank; 2017. Available from: https://openknowledge.worldbank.org/handle/10986/25880

[57] Rhodes RAW. Understanding governance: Ten years on. Organization Studies. 2007;**28**(8):1243-1264

[58] United Nations Economic and Social Commission for Asia and the Pacific. What is Good Governance? Bangkok, Thailand: United Nations; 2009. p. 3

[59] Gribble JN, Bremner J. Achieving a demographic dividend. Population Bulletin. 2012;**16**

[60] Argaw MD, Desta BF, Muktar SA, Abera WS, Beshir IA, Otoro IA, et al. Comparison of maternal and child health service performances following a leadership, management, and governance intervention in Ethiopia: A propensity score matched analysis. BMC Health Services Research. 2021;**21**(1):862

[61] Fernandez CSP, Noble CC, Garman L. A qualitative analysis of individual leadership behaviors among participants in the maternal and child health public health leadership institute. Maternal and Child Health Journal. 2021;**25**(7):1094-1101

[62] Fernandez CSP, Noble CC, Garman L. A qualitative analysis of maternal and child health public health leadership institute (MCH PHLI) leaders: Assessing the application of leadership skills at the "Others" and "Wider Community" levels of the MCH leadership competencies 4.0. Maternal and Child Health Journal. 2021;**25**(9):1437-1446

[63] McGrath ER, Bacso DR, Andrews JG, Rice SA. Intentional interprofessional

leadership in maternal and child health. Leadership in Health Services. 2018;**32**(2):212-225

[64] Umble KE, Powis L, Coffey AM, Margolis L, Mullenix A, Fatima H, et al. Developing state leadership in maternal and child health: Process evaluation findings from a work-based learning model for leadership development. Maternal and Child Health Journal. 2022. DOI: 10.1007/s10995-022-03444-z

[65] Buakhai P, Rithpho P. Reflections of positive experiences in midwifery and nursing of maternal-newborn education in Thailand: Lessons learned from naresuan university. Journal of Health and Caring Sciences. 2019;**1**(2):110-117

[66] Preker AS, Cotlear D, Kwon S, Atun R, Avila C. Universal health care in middle-income countries: Lessons from four countries. Journal of Global Health. 2021;**11**:16004

[67] Union A. Africa Heath Strategy 2016-2030. Addis Ababa; 2016. p. 33

[68] Kudamatsu M. Has democratization reduced infant mortality in sub-Saharan Africa? Evidence from micro data. Journal of the European Economic Association. 2012;**10**(6):1294-1317

[69] Diop N, Kamal M, Naffa S, Renaud M, Sinzinkayo F. African leadership and international collaboration to address global health challenges: Learnings from the Innovating for Maternal and Child Health in Africa (IMCHA) initiative. African Journal of Reproductive Health. 2021;**25**(3s). Available from: https://ajrh.info/index.php/ajrh/article/view/2797

[70] Izugbara CO, Kabiru CW, Amendah D, Dimbuene ZT, Donfouet HPP, Atake EH, et al. "It takes more than a fellowship program": Reflections on capacity strengthening for health systems research in sub-Saharan Africa. BMC Health Services Research. 2017;**17**(2):696

[71] Marston C, Cleland J. Relationships between contraception and abortion: A review of the evidence. International Family Planning Perspectives. 2003;**29**(1):6

[72] World Health Organization. World Malaria Report 2019. Geneva, Switzerland; 2019. p. 232 Report No.: Licence: CC BY-NC-SA 3.0 IGO. Available from: https://www.who.int/publications/i/item/9789241565721

Chapter 8

# Endothelial Dysfunction and Intestinal Barrier Injury in Preterm Infants with Perinatal Asphyxia

*Huseynova Saadat Arif, Panakhova Nushaba Farkhad, Orujova Pusta Ali, Hajiyeva Nurangiz Nizami, Hajiyeva Adila Sabir, Mukhtarova Sevinj Nabi and Agayeva Gulnaz Telman*

## Abstract

Perinatal asphyxia is one of the most frequent causes of perinatal morbidity, accounting for approximately 23% of neonatal deaths worldwide. Fetuses that suffer from hypoxia-ischemia are at high risk of developing multiorgan dysfunction, including the gut. Hypoxie-induced gut injury may result in adverse clinical outcomes, such as feeding intolerance and necrotizing enterocolitis. Increased permeability and subsequently an enhanced entry of bacteria and endotoxins into the systemic circulation can contribute to endotoxin aggression and further trigger numerous diseases. The aim of study is to investigate the effect of perinatal asphyxia on the integrity of the intestinal barrier and the state of antiendotoxin immunity. The study included preterm neonates exposed to perinatal asphyxia, who were comparable with non-asphyxiated infants. The concentrations of intestinal mucosa barrier injury markers (intestinal fatty acid binding protein, liver fatty acid protein, lipopolysaccharide binding protein), neurospecific proteins (neurospesific enolase, NR-2 antibodies), and also endothelial dysfunction markers (endothelin-1, nitric oxide) were determined in serum of included neonates on day of 1 and 7. The high risk of intestinal mucosal injury in newborn exposed to perinatal asphyxia decreases the level of antiendotoxic immunity and should be considered as an unfavorable factor for sepsis.

**Keywords:** perinatal asphyxia, endothelial function, brain injury, mucosal barrier, preterm infants

## 1. Introduction

The main pathophysiological change that develops in intestinal ischemia is damage to the epithelial integrity of the mucosa, leading to bacterial translocation, release of pro- and anti-inflammatory cytokines, activation of innate immunity dominated by pro-inflammatory effects, with the final manifestation of the process as intestinal perforation or fulminant sepsis [1, 2]. The progression of intestinal ischemia is combined with a paradoxical direction of oxygen flow in the villi from tissues to blood, which contributes to their hypoxia and can result in necrosis starting from the tops of the villi of the intestinal mucosa. In this case, enterocytes exfoliate from their own plate and into the intestinal lumen. One of the promising methods for assessing damage to intestinal epithelial cells is the determination of endogenous proteins of enterocytes in blood serum or urine [3]. These are low molecular weight proteins (14–15 kDa), fatty acid-binding proteins (FABPs), and bile acid-binding proteins. The intestinal form of FABP (I-FABP) is tissue-specific for the gut. I-FABP is localized to the tops of the villi in enterocytes and enters circulation when they are destroyed and is excreted from the body by the kidneys in a single passage, resulting in a half-life of 11 min. The concentration of this protein in the blood of healthy individuals does not usually exceed 2 ng/mL, but this increases rapidly after an episode of acute intestinal ischemia. Reisinger et al. found that the content of I-FABP in human and sheep intestinal villi depends on gestational age, and an increase in I-FABP content in blood occurs in parallel with gestational age, allowing its use as a marker to indicate intestinal maturity [4]. Given the particular importance of hypoxia in the pathogenesis of ulcerative necrotizing enterocolitis (NEC), the determination of I-FABP content is typically carried out to diagnose patients and determine the severity of this condition. In particular, in a study by Guthmann, concentrations of I-FABP and hepatic FABP (L-FABP) were determined in healthy preterm newborns and in preterm infants with ulcerative NEC. An increase in the I-FABP concentration was found in end-stage ulcerative NEC, while the concentration of L-FABP was significantly increased only in newborns with suspected ulcerative NEC. Tentatively, the identified changes may be useful for the early diagnosis of ulcerative NEC in newborns [5]. Mannoia K. et al. found high concentrations of I-FABP in urine collected in the first 60 h of life from preterm infants who subsequently developed ulcerative NEC with the onset of enteral nutrition. The authors proposed the use of this protein for early ulcerative NEC detection in newborns who are at high risk of developing it, allowing for timely preventive measures [6].

Intestinal mucosa and submucosa layers are characterized by an intensive blood supply, which is due to their high demand for oxygen to support the processes of hydrolysis and absorption of substances as well as the constant need to renew enterocytes exfoliating into the intestinal cavity [7]. At the same time, the consistency of the protective properties of the mucous barrier of the large intestine is determined by the level of expression of epithelial mucins and their properties. Active expression of mucins by the epithelium of the gastrointestinal tract (GIT) is accompanied by the formation of a high-molecular viscoelastic layer, which is a protective barrier between the surface of the mucous membrane and the cavity contents of the GIT. According to modern concepts, MUC2, MUC4, MUC3, and MUC17 are synthesized both in the small intestine and in the proximal and distal parts of the large intestine. The localization of mucins in the unchanged mucosa of the GIT coincides with the distribution of trefoil peptides expressed by goblet cells. Intestinal trefoil factor (ITF) together with mucins performs protective and regenerative functions, participating in the formation of the gastrointestinal barrier. Due to its compact structure, ITF is extremely resistant to acid attack, proteolytic degradation, and thermal degradation. Excessive synthesis of this substance occurs at sites of GIT damage, such as peptic ulcers or damage caused be inflammatory bowel disease. Patients with these pathologies have an elevated level of ITF in the blood serum. Lin J. et al., studying the level of ITF in neonatal meconium, found no difference in ITF content depending on birth weight [8]. Louis N.A. et al. argued that hypoxia has an inducing effect on the expression of

MUC3 and ITF in the intestinal mucosa, performing a protective function in oxygen-deficient conditions [9].

It has been proven that the violation of intestinal perfusion is accompanied by an increase in intestinal permeability, which may be due to the extensive death of the intestinal mucosa. The hyperoxia that occurs during the period of reperfusion, stimulating the processes of free radical oxidation and neutrophil chemotaxis, exacerbates inflammatory processes in the intestinal wall [10]. Another reason for the death of the intestinal mucosa may be severe endotoxemia. Endotoxins (lipopolysaccharides (LPS)), by stimulating the release of inflammatory mediators from macrophages and neutrophils, ultimately lead to an imbalance of pro- and anti-inflammatory responses, the occurrence of excessive systemic inflammation, and damage to the intestinal mucosal barrier [11].

Increased intestinal permeability describes an increase in the ability of substances to pass through the intestinal wall. Several non-invasive methods of examining intestinal permeability have been described. These methods can be divided into the following three groups: active direct, passive, and indirect. The "active" assessment of barrier function is based on the hypothesis that under physiological conditions, orally administered large molecules are unable to cross the intestinal wall. In the case of increased permeability, such samples cross the intestinal barrier and enter the bloodstream with subsequent detection in the urine after renal excretion. Absorption tests of water-soluble non-ionized compounds, such as lactulose, mannitol, and ethylenediaminetetraacetic acid, are most commonly used for this purpose. The "passive" assessment of the state of the intestinal barrier is based on the hypothesis that the intracavitary components of the intestine are translocated into the bloodstream with a decrease in its barrier function. Determination of the level of LPS of the outer membrane of Gram-negative bacteria (endotoxins) as well as measurement of the fermentation product D-lactate are the most commonly used tests for monitoring passive permeability. An indirect way to assess the translocation of bacterial products is to measure serum LPS-binding protein (LBP) levels and antibody levels in the endotoxin cortex.

LBP got its name from its ability to form a complex with LPS. LPS, which is the main component of the cell wall of Gram-negative microorganisms, is found in small amounts in the blood of healthy organisms and helps to maintain the protective mechanisms of innate immunity. LBP initiates the launch of a complex response cascade of the receptor complex with LPS, which consists of the recognition, binding, and transport of LPS and the enhancement of the infection danger signal [12]. The cascade of successive LPS-LRP reactions with receptor structures that recognize pathogen-associated samples initiates an intracellular signaling cascade, which, in turn, activates the nuclear transcription factor NF-kB with increased expression of pro-inflammatory mediators and rapid elimination of the infectious agent from the body. With excessive intake of LPS into the bloodstream and insufficient antiendotoxin protection, endotoxin aggression can develop. Synthesis of LBP mainly occurs in the liver with release into the blood after glycosylation with a molecular weight of 58–60 kDa [13].

Juli M. Richter et al. in experimental studies on rats established a dose-dependent effect of LBP on the processes of neonatal enterocyte migration and wound healing of the intestinal wall induced by LPS. Studies have found that a high concentration of LBP, as opposed to a normal concentration, suppresses the release of cytokines and improves survival after exposure of rats to LPS from *Escherichia coli* [14].

Present chapter describes the results of prospective clinical trial about the role of perinatal asphyxia in formation of intestinal barrier dysfunction. The study conducted by the neonatology research group of Azerbaijan Medical University and involved 240 preterm newborns with the risk of perinatal hypoxic encephalopathy with a gestational age of 32–36 weeks. Group 1 included newborns who experienced asphyxia during childbirth, and Group 2 included newborns with chronic intrauterine hypoxia but a relatively favorable course during the intranatal period. The Control group consisted of apparently healthy premature newborns. The levels of intestinal ischemia and neuronal injury makers were detected with standard ELISA method.

Chronic intrauterine hypoxia was determined on the basis of dopplerographic and cardiotocographic examination of the fetus. Asphyxia was diagnosed according to the guidelines of the American Academy of Pediatrics based on an Apgar score of <7 taken in the first 30 min of life [15]. Gestational age was determined by the date of the last menstruation of the mother, ultrasound examination of fetometric parameters. The severity of hypoxic–ischemic encephalopathy was determined based on the Sarnat score [16]. An ultrasound examination of the brain was performed on the third day of life using transducers with a frequency of 5 and 7.5 MHz. The degree of intraventricular hemorrhage was determined according to the Papile classification [17]. The exclusion criteria were a gestational age of <32 weeks, congenital malformations, and manifest forms of TORCH infections.

## 2. The impact of perinatal asphyxia on the intestinal barrier function

Involvement in the pathological process of the GIT is a logical outcome of severe hypoxic injury [18]. The causes of damage to the GIT are hemodynamic disorders, including regional disorders that involve a decrease in blood circulation in the mesenteric arteries in the first few minutes of life in newborns who have undergone asphyxia [19, 20]. The urinary concentration of the intestinal ischemia marker in newborns exposed to acute asphyxia in labor at 7–10 days old is significantly different from that of both healthy infants and newborns of Group 2 ($p_{1-3} = 0.05$: reliability of the difference for 1–3 days, $p_{7-10} = 0.005$: reliability of the difference for 7–10 days) (**Figure 1**).

Due to damage to the intestinal mucosa, failure of defense mechanisms, and overgrowth of Gram-negative intestinal flora, colonizing bacteria enter the mesenteric lymph nodes and systemic circulation. Impaired gut barrier function, even in the absence of bacteremia, leads to portal and systemic endotoxemia, which triggers a hypermetabolic and immunoinflammatory response. As can be seen from **Figure 1**, in Group 2 newborns, ischemia of the intestinal wall was accompanied by a high concentration of a marker of antiendotoxin immunity. In infants in Group 1, the level of LBP was significantly low compared to that in Group 2 infants, which indicated the failure of immune defense mechanisms in acute asphyxia that developed against the background of chronic intrauterine hypoxia ($p_{1-3} = 0.04$: reliability of the difference for 1–3 days, $p_{7-10} = 0.042$: reliability of the difference for 7–10 days). It should be noted that Juli M. Richter et al. indicated an improvement in the processes of regeneration of the intestinal epithelium susceptible to LPS attack after intraperitoneal administration of LBP at high concentrations [14]. The physiological increase in the level of this marker in newborns of the Control group was due to intestinal colonization, contact with bacteria, components of the colostrum, or postpartum maturation of the liver of newborns [21, 22].

As shown in **Figure 2**, the concentration of ITF, which stabilizes intestinal mucus and attenuates damage to the intestinal barrier, in newborns of Group 1 exceeded that of healthy newborns and infants of Group 2 (37.3 ± 9.0 ng/mL: subgroup

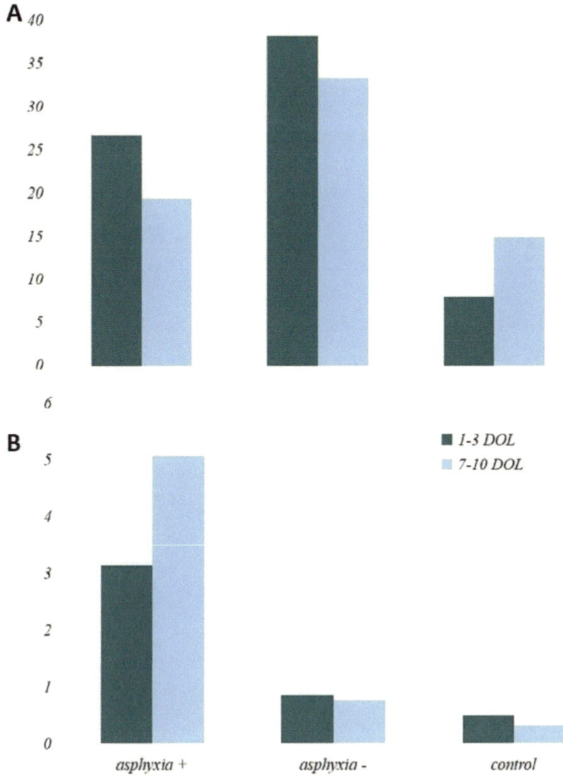


**Figure 1.**
*The levels of serum LBP (A, ng/ml) and urine IFABP (B, ng/ml) of newborns in asphyxia in 1–3 and 7–10 days of life (DOL).*

asphyxia +, 15.58 ± 3.7 ng/mL: subgroup asphyxia –, $p_{1-3}$ = 0.05: reliability of the difference for 1–3 days). Despite the decrease in the concentration of this marker in dynamics, the concentration continued to exceed the indicators of the other two groups (20.1 ± 2.5 ng/mL: subgroup asphyxia +, 7.2 ± 4.8 ng/mL: subgroup asphyxia –, $p_{7-10}$ = 0/064: reliability of the difference for 7–10 days). According to Nancy A. Louis, the expression of HIF-1 under hypoxic conditions and early reperfusion after ischemia triggers a physiological response characterized by the activation of functional mucus proteins, such as trefoil factor and P glycoprotein, aimed at preventing inflammatory processes in the intestine [9, 23].

At the same time, the level of secreted mucin does not increase in response to hypoxia (**Figure 2**); on the contrary, in newborns exposed to acute hypoxia, the level of Mucin-2 (MUC2), although not significantly, was slightly lower than that in the other two groups (14.83 ± 9.0 ng/mL: subgroup asphyxia +, 16.82 ± 0.7 ng/mL: subgroup asphyxia –, $p_{1-3}$ = 0.16: reliability of the difference for 1–3 days, 10.58 ± 1.4 ng/mL: subgroup asphyxia +, 16.67 ± 1.4 ng/mL: subgroup asphyxia –, $p_{7-10}$ = 0.06: reliability of the difference for 7–10 days).

The level of plasma L-FABP in newborns prone to asphyxia was 1.5 times lower than that in newborns of Group 2 (**Figure 2**) and did not differ from that of the Control group (1.94 ± 0.5 ng/mL: subgroup asphyxia +, 2.94 ± 0.5 ng/mL: subgroup asphyxia – for 1–3 days, 1.34 ± 0.2 ng/mL: subgroup asphyxia +, 2.15 ± 0.3 ng/mL: subgroup asphyxia – for 7–10 days). In general, on days 1–3 and 7–10, no significant

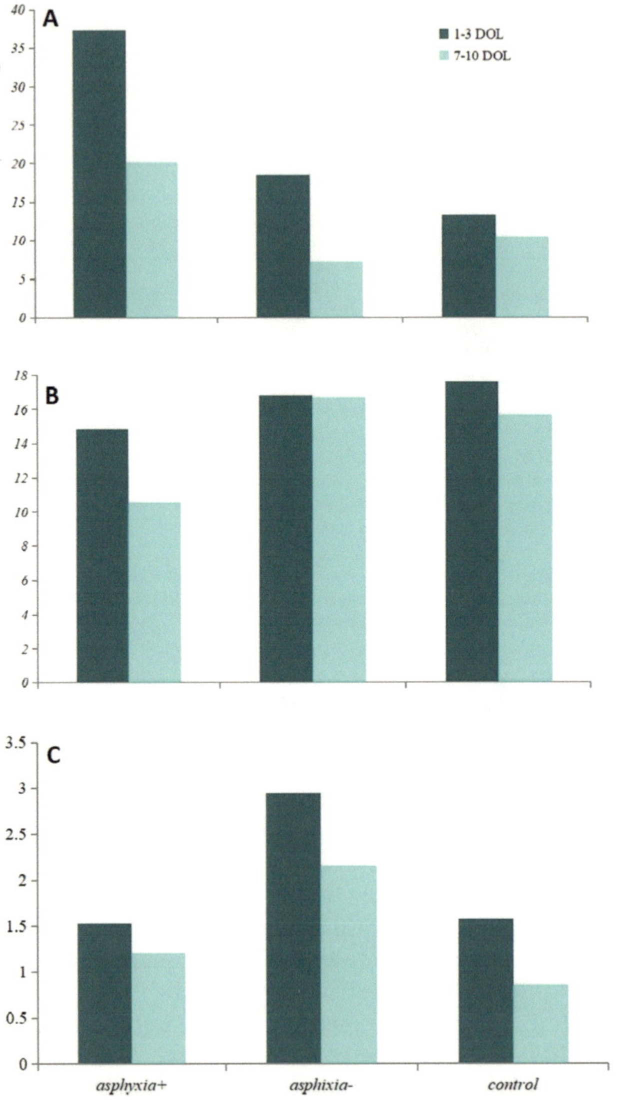


**Figure 2.**
*The levels of ITF (A, ng/ml), MUC2 (B, ng/ml), and LFABP (C, ng/ml) in peripheral blood of newborns in asphyxia in 1–3 and 7–10 days of life (DOL).*

differences in relation to this indicator were found between the studied groups ($p_{1-3}$ = 0.172: value of difference for 1–3 days, $p_{7-10}$ = 0.098: reliability of the difference for 7–10 days).

Despite chronic hypoxia and weakness of autoregulation in the GIT and kidneys compared to other vascular pools, the liver, due to its blood supply from two sources, is better protected from hypoxia and ischemia. Thus, newborns with a low birth weight prone to acute birth asphyxia are characterized by a high detection rate of organ and systemic disorders of posthypoxic origin. The obtained results showed that perinatal hypoxia initiates processes leading to an increase in the permeability of cell membranes, neuronal death due to necrosis or apoptosis, disruption of the integrity of the blood–brain barrier structure, and entry of brain antigens into systemic circulation, stimulating the immune system to produce antibrain antibodies. Disorders of the systemic and peripheral circulation, disorders of oxygen uptake, and delivery to tissues accompanying perinatal asphyxia develop a number of pathophysiological and pathobiochemical cascades that lead to secondary damage to the intestines and kidney parenchyma.

## 3. Endothelial dysfunction and the formation of the functional status of the intestinal mucosal barrier in newborns with a low birth weight prone to perinatal hypoxia

Endothelial dysfunction against the background of hypoxia and ischemia is accompanied by central nervous system lesions as well as dysfunctions of peripheral organs and systems [24, 25]. Visceral hypoperfusion is accompanied by the activation of indigenous microflora, damaging the immature intestinal barrier. Loss of the intestinal barrier can lead, due to the resorption of endotoxins, bacteria, and other substances, to systemic inflammatory reaction syndrome, remote organ damage, and multiple organ failure [26]. Considering the above, the purpose of this study was to determine the effect of endothelial dysfunction on the levels of markers, reflecting the functional state of the digestive system in newborns with a low birth weight with perinatal hypoxia.

Neurons and glial cells, whose need for energy supply is higher than that of all other cells of the body, are the first to suffer under conditions of oxygen deficiency. In this study, the biochemical marker of the destruction of nerve cells and the permeability of the blood–brain barrier in newborns of Group 1 and 2 significantly exceeded the indicators of the Control group on days 1–3 and 7–10 of life (**Figure 3**). The highest values of this marker are typical for newborns prone to acute birth asphyxia. Degradation of NMDA receptors as a result of neurotoxicity, assessed by the level of antibodies to NR2, in newborns of Group 1 significantly differed from the indicators of the Control group

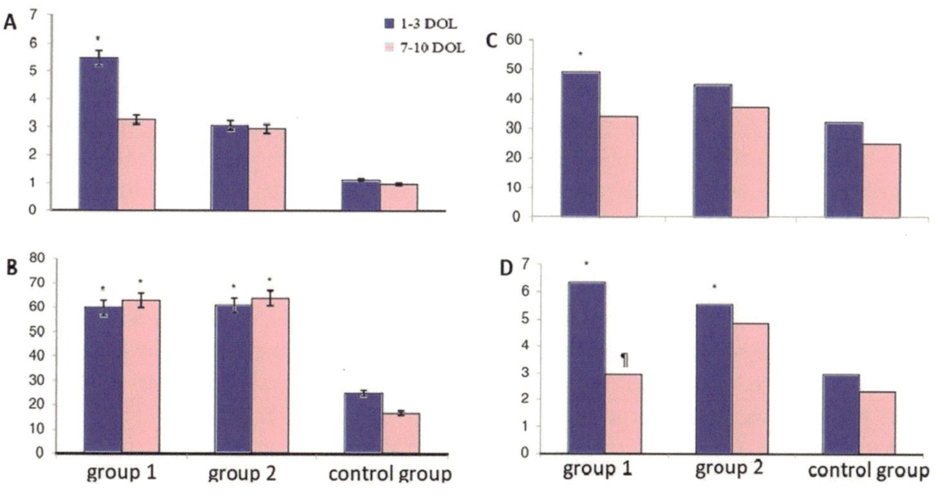


**Figure 3.**
*The blood concentrations of NR2 (A, ng/ml), NSE (B, ng/ml), NO (C, ng/ml), and ET-1 (D, ng/ml) in infants with hypoxic–ischemic encephalopathy in 1–3 and 7–10 days of life (DOL). *Significance of difference in comparison with control infants; significance of difference in comparison with second group.*

for both the first and second measurements, although a significant difference between Groups 1 and 2 was not found. This may be due, on the one hand, to the peculiarities of the immune response of immature newborns, which significantly predominate in the group subject to acute birth asphyxia. On the other hand, a longer period of time is required for the formation of ischemia foci and the accumulation of antibodies to glutamate receptors. The dynamics of the content of vasoregulatory markers in the peripheral blood in the studied groups are also shown in **Figure 3**. Both Group 1 and 2 were characterized by high concentrations of NO, while a significant difference in relation to this indicator was found between Group 1 and the Control group. Despite the level of endothelin-1 being initially high in both groups subject to chronic intrauterine hypoxia, in the group of newborns with acute asphyxia, the content of this marker sharply decreased toward the end of the perinatal period.

Violation of the vasoregulatory function of the vascular endothelium, manifested by a low level of endothelin-1 against the background of a high concentration of NO, in chronic intrauterine hypoxia complicated by acute birth asphyxia, being a causative factor in reducing blood pressure, leads to tissue ischemia. Visceral hypoperfusion in children with perinatal asphyxia is the leading cause of abdominal complications. Ischemia triggers a vicious circle of damage to the gastrointestinal mucosa and serves as a trigger for the formation of multiple organ failure [27]. The level of the intestinal ischemia marker I-FABP in newborns of Group 1 and 2 did not significantly exceed that of the Control group in the first days of life; however, it almost doubled in dynamics and differed significantly from the level of healthy infants (**Figure 4**).

Due to damage to the intestinal mucosa, failure of defense mechanisms, and overgrowth of Gram-negative intestinal flora, colonizing bacteria penetrate the mesenteric lymph nodes and systemic circulation (bacterial translocation) [28]. Violation of the intestinal barrier function, even in the absence of bacteremia, leads to portal and systemic endotoxemia, which serves as a trigger for a hypermetabolic and immunoinflammatory response [29]. The level of plasma L-FABP in newborns subject to asphyxia was 1.5 times lower than that in newborns of Group 2 and did not differ from that in the Control group. In general, on days 1–3 and 7–10, no significant differences in relation to this indicator were found between the studied groups. Despite chronic hypoxia and weakness of autoregulation in the GIT and liver compared to other vascular pools, the liver, due to its blood supply being from two sources, is better protected from hypoxia and ischemia. As can be seen in **Figure 4**, in newborns of Group 2, ischemia of the intestinal wall was accompanied by a high concentration of the marker of antiendotoxin immunity. In children in Group 1, the level of LBP was significantly lower than that in Group 2, indicating the failure of immune defense mechanisms in acute asphyxia that developed against the background of chronic intrauterine hypoxia.

Juli M. Richter et al. indicated an improvement in the processes of regeneration of the intestinal epithelium susceptible to LPS attack after intraperitoneal administration of LBP at high concentrations [14]. The physiological increase in the level of this marker in newborns of the Control group was due to intestinal colonization, contact with bacteria, colostrum components, or postpartum maturation of the liver [30]. The concentration of ITF, which stabilizes intestinal mucus and attenuates damage to the intestinal barrier, in newborns of Group 1 exceeded that of healthy newborns and infants in Group 2 (**Figure 5**). This difference was significant only for the Control group. Despite the decrease in this marker in dynamics, its content continued to exceed the indicators of the other two groups. According to Nancy A. Louis, HIF1 expression under hypoxic conditions and early reperfusion after ischemia trigger a

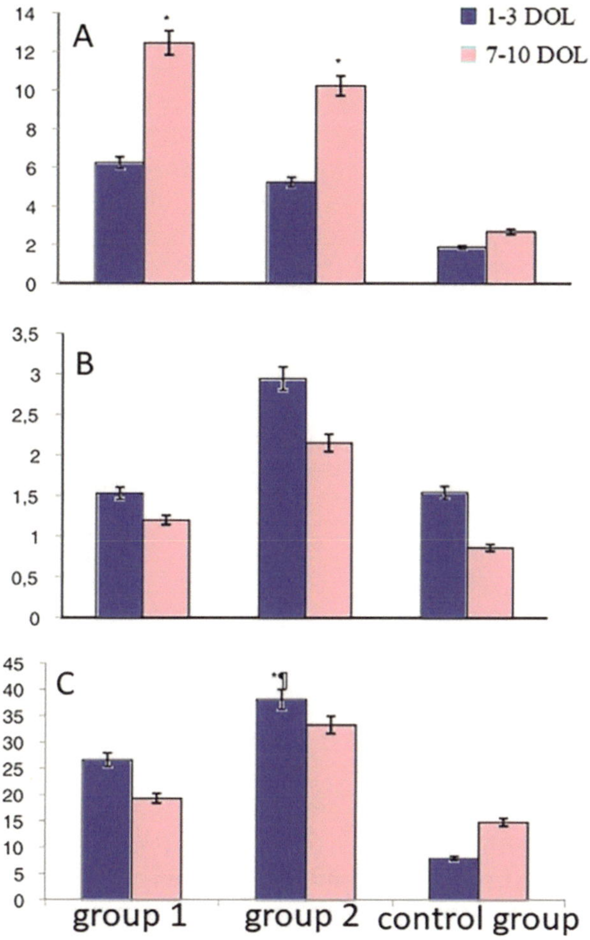


**Figure 4.**
*The blood concentrations of IFABP (A, ng/ml), LFABP (B, ng/ml), and LBP (C, ng/ml) in infants with hypoxic–ischemic encephalopathy in 1–3 and 7–10 days of life (DOL). *Significance of difference in comparison with control infants; significance of difference in comparison with group 1.*

physiological response characterized by the activation of functional mucus proteins, such as trefoil factor and P glycoprotein, aimed at preventing inflammatory processes in the intestine [23, 31]. At the same time, the level of secreted mucin does not increase in response to hypoxia. On the contrary, in this study, in newborns exposed to acute hypoxia, the level of MUC2, although not significantly, was somewhat lower than that of the other two groups.

Thus, newborns with a low birth weight subject to acute birth asphyxia are characterized by a high detection rate of organ and systemic disorders of posthypoxic origin. The results obtained showed that perinatal hypoxia initiated processes leading to an increase in the permeability of cell membranes, neuron death due to necrosis and/or apoptosis, disruption of the integrity of the blood–brain barrier structure, and entry of brain antigens into the systemic circulation, stimulating the immune system to produce antibrain antibodies. Involvement in the pathological process of the GIT is a logical outcome of severe hypoxic injury. The cause of damage to the digestive system is hemodynamic disturbances as a result of endothelial dysfunction, including

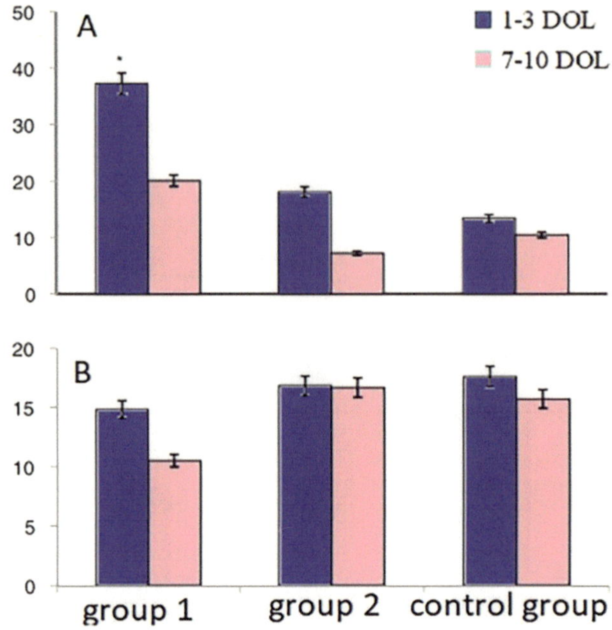


**Figure 5.**
*The blood concentrations of ITF (A, ng/ml) and MUC-2 (B, ng/ml) in infants with hypoxic–ischemic encephalopathy in 1–3 and 7–10 days of life (DOL). *Significance of difference in comparison with control infants.*

regional dysfunction with a decrease in blood circulation in the mesenteric arteries in the first minutes of life in newborns who have experienced asphyxia. Disorders of the systemic and peripheral circulation as well as disorders of oxygen uptake and delivery to tissues accompanying perinatal asphyxia result in the development of a number of pathophysiological and pathobiochemical cascades, leading to secondary damage to the GIT.

## Author details

Huseynova Saadat Arif[1], Panakhova Nushaba Farkhad[2,3]*, Orujova Pusta Ali[2], Hajiyeva Nurangiz Nizami[2], Hajiyeva Adila Sabir[3], Mukhtarova Sevinj Nabi[2] and Agayeva Gulnaz Telman[2,3]

1 Scientific Research Institute of Obstetrics and Gynecology, Baku, Azerbaijan

2 Azerbaijan Medical University, Baku, Azerbaijan

3 Scientific Research Institute of Pediatrics After Name K. Farajova, Baku, Azerbaijan

*Address all correspondence to: nushaba2009@yandex.ru

## References

[1] Emami C, Chokshi N, Wang J, et al. Role of interleukin-10 in the pathogenesis of necrotizing enterocolitis. American Journal of Surgery. 2012;**203**(4):428-435

[2] Grishin A, Bowling J, Bell B, et al. Roles of nitric oxide and intestinal mikrobiota in the pathogenesis of necrotizing enterocolitis. Journal of Pediatric Surgeory. 2016;**51**(1):13-17

[3] Alsina M, Martín-Ancel A, Alarcon-Allen A, et al. The severity of hypoxic-ischemic encephalopathy correlates with multiple organ dysfunction in the hypothermia era. Neonatal Intensive Care. 2017;**18**(3):234-240

[4] Reisinger KW, Elst M, Derikx JPM, et al. Intestinal fatty acid–binding protein: A possible marker for gut maturation. Pediatric Research. 2014;**76**(3):261-268. DOI:10.1038/pr.2014.89

[5] Guthmann F, Borchers T, Wolfrum C, et al. Plasma concentration of intestinal- and liver-FABP in neonates suffering from necrotizing enterocolitis and in healthy preterm. Molecular and Cellular Biochemistry. 2002;**239**(1-2):227-234

[6] Mannoia K, Boskovic D, Slater L, et al. Necrotizing enterocolitis is associated with neonatal intestinal injury. Journal of Pediatric Surgery. 2001;**46**(1):81-85

[7] Shafizadeh T. Mucus degradation and gut microbes: Maintaining gut barrier function in the preterm infant. Neonatal Intensive Care. 2018;**31**(3):21-22

[8] Lin J, Nadroo A, Chen W, et al. Ontogeny and prenatal expression of trefoil factor 3/ITF in the human intestine. Early Human Development. 2003;**71**(2):103-109

[9] Panakhova NF, Hajiyeva AS, Huseynova SA, Hasanov SS, Hajiyeva NN. The relationship between intestinal protective markers and serum Endotheiln-1 concentrations in low birth weight infants with hypoxic-ischemic encephalopathy. International Journal of Pharmaceutical Sciences and Research. 2017;**8**(7):2832-2838

[10] Ricardo-da-Silva FY, Fantozzi ET, Rodrigues-Garbin S, et al. Estradiol prevented intestinal ischemia and reperfusion-induced changes in intestinal permeability and motility in male rats. Clinics. 2021;**76**:e2683. DOI:10.6061/clinics/2021/e2683

[11] Cui Y, Wang Q, Sun R, et al. Astragalus membranaceus (Fisch.) Bunge repairs intestinal mucosal injury induced by LPS in mice. BMC Complementary and Alternative Medicine. 2018;**18**:230. DOI:10.1186/s12906-018-2298-2

[12] Gutsmann T, Müller M, Carroll S, et al. Dual role of lipopolysaccharide (LPS)-binding protein in neutralization of LPS and enhancement of LPS-induced activation of mononuclear cells. Infection and Immunity. 2001;**69**(11):6942-6950

[13] Abdou S, Ramada K, Abumourad L, et al. Biocompatibility and gene expression associated with streptococcus infection in myocarditis. International Journal of Genetic Engineering. 2012;**2**(1):1-11

[14] Richter J, Schanbacher B, Huang H, et al. LPS-binding protein enables intestinal epithelial restitution despite LPS exposure. Journal of Pediatric Gastroenterology and Nutrition. 2012;**54**(5):639-644

[15] Chen ZL, He RZ, Peng Q, et al. Clinical study on improving the diagnostic criteria for neonatal asphyxia. Zhonghua Er Ke Za Zhi. 2006;**44**:167-172

[16] Sarnat H, Sarnat M. Neonatal encephalopathy following fetal distress: A clinical and electroencephalographic study. Archives of Neurology. 1976;**33**:695-706

[17] Papile L, Burstein J, Burstein R. Incidence and evolution of the subependymal intraventricular hemorrhage: A study of infants with weights less than 1500 grams. The Journal of Pediatrics. 1978;**92**:529-534

[18] Choi Y. Necrotizing enterocolitis in newborns: Update in pathophysiology and newly emerging therapeutic strategies. Korean Journal of Pediatrics. 2014;**57**(12):505-513

[19] Bennet L, Quaedackers JSL, Gunn AJ, et al. The effect of asphyxia on superior mesenteric artery blood flow in the premature sheep fetus. Journal of Pediatric Surgery. 2000;**35**(1):34-40

[20] Whitehouse J, Riggle K, Purpi D, et al. The protective role of intestinal alkaline phosphatase in necrotizing enterocolitis. The Journal of Surgical Research. 2010;**163**:7

[21] Richter J, Schanbacher B, Huang H, et al. LPS-binding protein enables intestinal epithelial restitution despite LPS exposure. Journal of Pediatric Gastroenterology and Nutrition. 2012;**54**(5):639-644

[22] Orlikowsky TW, Trug C, Neunhoeffer F. Lipopolysaccharide-binding protein in noninfected neonates and those with suspected early-onset bacterial infection. Journal of Perinatology. 2006;**26**:115-119

[23] Louis N, Hamilton K, Canny G, et al. Selective induction of mucin-3 by hypoxia in intestinal epithelia. Journal of Cellular Biochemistry. 2006;**99**(6):1616-1627

[24] Kadhim H, Khalifa M, Deltenre P, et al. Molecular mechanisms of cell death in periventricular leukomalacia. Neurology. 2006;**67**:293-299

[25] Huseynova S, Panakhova N, Orujova P, et al. Altered endothelial nitric oxide synthesis in preterm and small for gestational age infants. Pediatrics International. 2015;**2**:269-275

[26] Balzan S, Quadros CA, de Cleva R, et al. Bacterial translocation: Overview of mechanisms and clinical impact. Journal of Gastroente rology and Hepatology. 2007;**22**:464-471

[27] Blikslager AT. Life in the gut without oxygen: Adaptive mechanisms and inflammatory bowel disease. Gastroenterology. 2008;**134**:346-348

[28] Boston VE. Necrotising enterocolitis and localised intestinal perforation: Different diseases or ends of a spectrum of pathology. Pediatric Surgery International. 2006;**6**:477-484

[29] Berman L, Moss R. Necrotizing enterocolitis: An update. Seminars in Fetal & Neonatal Medicine. 2011;**16**:145-150

[30] Turner MA, Power S, Emmerson AJ. Gestational age and the C reactive protein response. Archives of Disease in Childhood. Fetal and Neonatal Edition. 2004;**89**:272-273

[31] Louis N, Hamilton K, Shekels L, et al. Selective induction of Mucin3 by hypoxia in intestinal epithelia. FASEB. 2006;**6**:1616-1627

Chapter 9

# Diabetes in Pregnancy

*Olakunmi Ololade Ogunyemi, Oluwakemi Mary Agoyi-Awoniyi and Hassan Taiwo Yahaya*

## Abstract

Pregnancy is usually a joyous event for most women and their families in many cultures. However, in certain situations, this celebratory moment is marred by various maternal complications; chief among them is diabetes mellitus. Over eighty percent of diabetes in pregnancy is attributed to Gestational Diabetes Mellitus (GDM). Also, GDM presents a higher risk of affected mothers developing diabetes later in the future. There is a growing prevalence of GDM which necessitates the need for closer monitoring and more screening of pregnant women. This can be achieved by following set guidelines of countries and public health organisations to ensure safer pregnancies, safer deliveries, and healthier babies.

**Keywords:** gestational diabetes, diabetes in pregnancy, complications of pregnancy, pre-existing diabetes, management of GDM

## 1. Introduction

Pregnancy is usually a joyous event for most women and their families in many cultures. However, in certain situations, this celebratory moment is marred by various maternal complications; chief among them is diabetes mellitus.

Diabetes mellitus, also known as diabetes, is a metabolic disorder characterised by high blood glucose levels over a long period of time [1]. In pregnant women, it manifests as either gestational diabetes mellitus (GDM) or pre-existing diabetes [2]. Gestational diabetes mellitus (GDM) is defined as glucose intolerance of variable degree that is first discovered during pregnancy [3], while pre-existing diabetes is glucose intolerance existing before pregnancy.

Diabetes in pregnancy is associated with a number of poor outcomes during the pregnancy period, during childbirth, and the immediate postpartum period [2]. Infants of mothers with pre-existing diabetes mellitus also experience double the risk of serious injury at birth, triple the likelihood of caesarean delivery and quadruple the incidence of new-born intensive care unit (NICU) admission [4].

In this chapter, we'll be exploring the prevalence of diabetes in pregnancy, the body's adaptation to pregnancy, the pathophysiology of diabetes in pregnancy, associated complications, diagnostic criteria for GDM and PDM, the management of this condition, and recommendations to reduce its prevalence.

## 1.1 Epidemiology

Statistics show that about 87–90% of diabetes in pregnancy is GDM, whereas 10–13% is pre-existing diabetes [5]. Further data also shows that diabetes complicates 2–45% of pregnancies across the globe, depending on the region, population characteristics, and diagnostic criteria [6–8].

## 1.2 How the body adapts to pregnancy

In pregnancy, a woman's body goes through significant anatomic and physiological changes to provide the support needed to nurture the growing foetus, while still maintaining normal body functions required for survival [9]. Some of these changes are due to hormonal production before conception. These changes then consolidate throughout the period of pregnancy, affecting every system and organ in the woman's body. For the majority of women who experience uncomplicated pregnancy, these changes are reversed following delivery. It is important to understand the normal physiologic adaptations of the body to pregnancy, so we can recognise when an abnormal occurrence comes into the picture. Although the major system affected by GDM is the endocrine system, it is still important to explore some of the changes in the other systems of the body. This is because hyperglycaemia can affect multiple body systems.

### *1.2.1 Cardiovascular changes in pregnancy*

Beginning in the first trimester, changes are seen in the cardiovascular system, with cardiac output increasing by 20% as early as the eighth week of gestation [10]. This is mediated primarily by peripheral vasodilation which produces a 25–30% fall in systemic vascular resistance. To compensate for this fall, the heart increases the cardiac output to around 40% throughout pregnancy. This is achieved by a mix of increased stroke volume and heart rate. There is also a compensatory increase in plasma volume to about 50%, with a lesser increase in the red blood cell mass, and a fall in platelet count [11]. Some of these changes also lead to a hypercoagulable state in pregnancy.

Some examination findings may include collapsing pulse and murmur which may be erroneously interpreted as pathological.

### *1.2.2 Renal*

There is a 40% fall in systemic vascular resistance by the sixth week of pregnancy which affects the renal vasculature. As a consequence of renal vasodilatation, renal plasma flow and glomerular filtration rate (GFR) both increase, compared to non-pregnant levels, by 40–65% and 50–85%, respectively [12].

### *1.2.3 Respiratory system*

The demand for oxygen increases significantly during pregnancy due to the increased metabolic rate [10].

### *1.2.4 Endocrine system*

Changes occur in the endocrine system across the adrenal and thyroid glands, and also across the metabolic processes of the body. There is a change in how the body metabolises glucose, protein and lipids. More details will be shed specifically on glucose metabolism further down in the chapter.

### 1.3 Pathophysiology of diabetes

Diabetes Mellitus develops majorly as a result of either defective insulin secretion from the beta cells of the pancreas or a defect in the insulin-sensitive cells which reduces the body's response to the available insulin [1]. A dysfunction in any of these two processes leads to abnormally high glucose levels.

#### *1.3.1 Glucose regulation in a healthy adult*

The human body utilises glucose as an immediate source of energy. The optimal level of glucose for proper body functioning is usually about 70–100 mg/dL [13]. Any value below or above this range constitutes a problem. Although the body can utilise other fuels, like protein and fat, as a source of energy, the breakdown of these alternative fuels creates ketoacids which makes the body acidic. This can lead to metabolic acidosis—which is a non-optimal state [14].

Regulation of glucose in the blood is largely carried out by the endocrine hormones in the pancreas via a process of continuous negative feedback loop. The main hormones involved in this process are insulin, glucagon, somatostatin and amylin. Insulin, formed in the beta cells of the pancreas, is the main hormone in this process and it lowers blood glucose levels. Conversely, Glucagon increases blood glucose levels. Somatostatin, produced by the pancreas's delta cells, helps balance insulin and glucagon levels, while the Delta cells of the pancreas help to balance the levels of insulin and glucagon. Amylin is the hormone that induces the feeling of fullness following a meal, thus preventing overeating.

For glucose to be utilised by the body, it is transported at a cellular level through the body tissues. This transportation is regulated by insulin which aids the diffusion rate of glucose into cells. After glucose enters the cell, it is converted to glucose-6-phosphate which can either be used immediately or be stored as glycogen.

#### *1.3.2 Glucose regulation during pregnancy*

As earlier explained, during a healthy pregnancy, a woman's body undergoes various physiological changes to meet the demands of the growing foetus in her womb. The adaptive change that is important for glucose metabolism occurs in the metabolic systems. During this period the insulin sensitivity of the woman's body varies to meet the requirements of pregnancy. In the early phase of gestation, insulin sensitivity is increased thus promoting the uptake of glucose into storage for the later part of pregnancy. As gestation progresses, there is a surge of several hormones including placental hormones, oestrogen, cortisol, placental growth hormone, placental lactogen, progesterone and leptin. This surge leads to a state of insulin resistance which elevates blood glucose levels. This insulin-resistant state leads to the endogenous production of glucose via the breakdown of protein and fats, further increasing the level of blood glucose. The glucose is transported to the foetus via the placenta to aid growth in-utero.

Some evidence shows that the maternal body compensates for this state of resistance through hypertrophy and hyperplasia of pancreatic beta-cells to produce more insulin. Placental hormones are important in this process as the maternal state of insulin sensitivity is reversed after a few days following the foetus and placenta delivery. Gestational Diabetes often occurs when there is an imbalance in this process.

### 1.4 Presentation and diagnostic criteria

Diabetes in pregnancy often presents with similar symptoms as diabetes in the rest of the population. These symptoms include increased thirst, increased urination, and increased appetite. However, these symptoms may either be absent in pregnancy or falsely attributed to pregnancy symptoms thus the diagnosis may be overlooked. Typically, diabetes in pregnancy goes undiagnosed until blood glucose is checked at antenatal visits.

It is important to note that pregnant women who are categorised as 'low-risk' do not require glucose testing. However, this category is limited to women who meet all the following criteria:

- Age lesser than 25 years.
- Normal weight before pregnancy.
- Member of an ethnic group with a low prevalence of GDM.
- No known history of diabetes in first-degree relatives.
- No personal history of abnormal glucose tolerance.
- No personal history of poor obstetric outcomes.

#### *1.4.1 Risk factors for DM*

There are certain factors that predispose pregnant women to a higher risk of GDM. Some of these include [15]:

1. Obesity, particularly severe obesity.
2. First-degree relatives living with type 2 DM.
3. Medical history of GDM, or delivery history of large for gestational age (LGA) infant.
4. Polycystic ovarian syndrome (PCOS).
5. Recurrent glycosuria positive result.

It should be noted that screening for GDM usually occurs between weeks 24–28—second or third trimester—of the gestational period. As such, high levels of glucose seen in the first trimester are often grouped as pre-pregnancy diabetes.

#### *1.4.2 Risk factors for GDM*

Pregnant women in this category are at a higher risk of developing GDM [15]:

1. Factors with the pregnant woman:
    - 35 years old or older;
    - overweight or obese prior to pregnancy;
    - personal history of impaired glucose tolerance;
    - Polycystic Ovarian Syndrome (PCOS)
2. A family history of diabetes
3. Abnormal pregnancy and/or delivery history:
    - unexplained foetal death, stillbirth or miscarriage;
    - foetal macrosomia;
    - foetal malformations;
    - polyhydramnios;
    - Gestational Diabetes Mellitus (GDM)
4. Conditions in present pregnancy:
    - large for gestational age;
    - polyhydramnios;
    - recurrent vulvovaginal candidiasis

#### *1.4.3 Diagnostic criteria*

Normal blood glucose levels range from 70 mg/dL (3.9 mmol/L) to 100 mg/dL (5.6 mmol/L). When the fasting blood glucose (FBG) is between 100 and 125 mg/dL (5.6–6.9 mmol/L), changes in lifestyle and monitoring glycaemia are recommended [13]. However, when the fasting blood glucose is 126 mg/dL (7 mmol/L) or higher on two separate occasions, a diagnosis of diabetes mellitus is made. The diagnostic standard cut-off point for diagnosing GDM is the 50-g Glucose Challenge Test with ≥7.8 mmol/L (140 mg/dl) as the cut-off point [15].

##### *1.4.3.1 Diagnosis of pregnancy complicated by DM*

Diagnosis for pregnancy complicated by DM can be diagnosed when any of these conditions exist [15]:

1. Glycosylated haemoglobin A1c (GHbA1c) ≥6.5%);
2. FPG ≥7.0 mmol/L (126 mg/dl);

3. 2-hour OGTT≥11.1 mmol/L (200 mg/dl);

4. Classic signs of hyperglycaemia or hyperglycaemic crises symptoms, meanwhile random plasma glucose ≥11.1 mmol/L (200 mg/dl)

*1.4.3.2 Diagnostic standard for GDM*

The Oral Glucose Tolerance Test (OGTT) is the gold standard for diagnosing GDM. The procedure involves eating a balanced diet containing at least 150 g of carbohydrates per day for 3 days prior to the test, which is followed by a period of fasting (no ingestion of any food) for 8 to 14 hours before the test.

The first blood sample is taken by 9 a.m. for measurement of the fasting blood glucose. After that, the patient is given a drink of 75-g glucose load (75-g glucose dissolved in 300 ml of water, consumed within 5 minutes). Following the ingestion of the glucose solution, blood samples are taken at 1 and 2-hour intervals to measure the blood glucose levels post-ingestion. During the waiting period, smoking, eating, or drinking any other fluids is prohibited.

*1.4.3.3 Diagnostic approaches****

The American College of Obstetricians and Gynaecologists recommends a two-step procedure for diagnosing GDM [3, 15]. If after 1 hour the blood glucose level is more than 7.8 mmol/L (140 mg/dL), a 100 g dose of glucose is given. The diagnosis of gestational diabetes is thus defined by a blood glucose level meeting or exceeding the cut-off values of at least two intervals:

- Before glucose intake (fasting): 5.3 mmol/L (95 mg/dL).
- 1 hour post-consumption of glucose solution: 10.0 mmol/L (180 mg/dL).
- 2 hours post-consumption of glucose solution: 8.6 mmol/L (155 mg/dL).
- 3 hours post-consumption of glucose solution: 7.8 mmol/L (140 mg/dL).

One-step approach: a diagnostic 75-g OGTT is performed at the 24th–28th week of gestation without the prior 50-g GCT screening. The one-step approach can be applied to high-risk pregnant women with GDM, or pregnant women not previously diagnosed with overt diabetes in well-conditioned medical institutions.

Two-step approach: measure FPG (step 1). If FPG ≥5.1 mmol/L, GDM can be diagnosed; if 4.4 mmol/L ≤ FPG <5.1 mmol/L, diagnostic 75-g OGTT (step 2) is followed to diagnose GDM. Or perform an initial screening by measuring the plasma or serum glucose concentration after a 50-g GCT (step 1) and perform a diagnostic OGTT (step 2) on that subset of women exceeding the glucose threshold value on the GCT. If 50-g GCT ≥11.1 mmol/L, FPG is performed to diagnose GDM; if the FPG value is normal, 75-g OGTT should be performed as soon as possible.

The cut-off points of glucose values of 75-g OGTT: 0 h, 5.1 mmol/L; 1 hour, 10.0 mmol/L; 2 hours, 8.5 mmol/L. The diagnosis of GDM can then be made when any one value is met or exceeded.

### 1.5 Complications of diabetes in pregnancy

Diabetes in pregnancy is associated with a number of complications in the mother and unborn foetus [16]. These complications can also extend beyond the duration of pregnancy. These complications can be divided into maternal complications and foetal complications.

#### *1.5.1 Maternal complications*

##### *1.5.1.1 Miscarriage*

Statistics show that women with PDM have a 9–14% rate of miscarriage [16]. Available data further suggests that there is a strong association between the degree of glycaemic control before pregnancy and the rate at which miscarriage occurs in women with PDM. In cases of more long-standing disease (>10 years) with poor control, the miscarriage rates can reach as high as 44%. Thankfully, the miscarriage rate normalises when glycaemic control is optimal.

##### *1.5.1.2 Progression to chronic diabetes mellitus*

In ideal conditions, GDM resolves after birth with glucose levels reverting to normal without further treatment. However, studies also show that women with GDM have a 16-year cumulative incidence of diabetes (60%) following the initial diabetic episode in pregnancy [17].

##### *1.5.1.3 Predisposition to other complications of pregnancy*

DM in pregnancy increases the risk of the mother developing other pregnancy complications such as pregnancy-induced hypertension, premature rupture of membranes, haemorrhage in the antepartum or postpartum period, and other possible complications [18]. Compared with women who do not have GDM, women with GDM have a higher risk of delivery by caesarean section.

#### *1.5.2 Foetal complications*

##### *1.5.2.1 Premature delivery*

Babies of mothers with GDM are at a higher risk of being born before the estimated due date, leading to premature delivery [19, 20].

##### *1.5.2.2 Problems at delivery*

These babies are also more likely to have several problems at birth ranging from macrosomia, small for date, foetal distress, hypoglycaemia, shoulder dystocia, birth asphyxia among others [19–21].

##### *1.5.2.3 Birth defects*

There is also a higher likelihood of such babies being born with birth defects and also having a higher risk of congenital heart diseases compared to the rest of the population [21].

#### 1.5.2.4 Obesity and DM in future

The effects of being born to a mother with GDM can very well linger beyond infancy and childhood, predisposing the individual to a risk of obesity and DM later in life.

## 2. Social determinants and effects of gestational diabetes outcomes

DM as a leading cause of NCD morbidity and mortality, especially in the vulnerable state of pregnancy has varying effects on the mother and developing child. Furthermore, as one of the most common metabolic disorders in pregnancy, its effects transcend into different aspects of maternal and neonatal health and wellbeing, including the public health space.

Some of these effects on mothers' health and physical wellbeing are hyperglycaemia, possible preeclampsia, high-risk delivery of a macrosomic baby; and if unmanaged, altered sensorium, eclampsia, obstetric problems and possible mortality. Likewise, different health complications of diabetes worsened by pregnancy include diabetic neuropathy, diabetic nephropathy, diabetic retinopathy, and diabetes-induced heart disease, i.e., cardiomyopathy, heart failure, ischemic heart disease and coronary heart disease. Some of these effects and complications are irreversible and take a strain on the financial and mental well-being of the pregnant woman and family involved. These complications can increase the direct or indirect cost of adequate care—with more time spent in the health care facility—which might have a poor prognosis among LSE women in rural areas, also worsening the maternal morbidity and mortality indices [21, 22].

Effects on foetal growth in-utero such as intrauterine growth retardation, and malformation of developing organs and systems in babies (also referred to as diabetic embryopathy), usually occurring in the first and second trimester, can lead to anxiety, depression and different types of miscarriage for the pregnant women. These foetal malformations are mostly found in the central nervous and cardiovascular systems, and sometimes with craniofacial defects. Common examples are Microcephaly, Meningomyelocele, Tetralogy of Fallot, persistent truncus arteriosus, Hypoplastic left or right heart syndrome, septal defects (Atrioventricular), Microphthalmia, Cleft lip/palate, Hemifacial microsomia and other neural tube defects [21].

Other effects surrounding delivery or occurring postnatally are preterm delivery, prematurity, low birth weight, other perinatal morbidities, neurodevelopmental abnormalities causing mental and psychomotor disabilities such as increased chances of Attention Deficit Hyperactivity Disorder (ADHD), gross and fine motor anomalies, learning difficulties (especially in speech and language), Autism Spectrum Disorder with possible brain damage, as well as perinatal mortality in the delivered neonates. The underlying metabolic processes that result in these effects could be associated with maternal hyperglycaemia causing increased oxidative stress, hypoxia, apoptosis, and epigenetic or metabolic changes in developing foetuses [21].

The socio-economic, health-economic, and psychosocial cost of these outcomes on the new mother, caregivers, healthcare professionals, family, society, and the entire population at large, is significantly wide and demanding with features of reduced productivity and preventable resource allocation for more judicious use. These also contribute to neonatal or under 5 morbidity and mortality figures. However, other cumulative factors that contribute to the actualization of these effects and their progress into complications for both mother and child vary from genetics to diet, or nutrition (especially breastfeeding infants for positive effect and development), compliance and environmental exposure [21].

## 3. Management

Management of GDM and PDM involves a variety of procedures. To start with, regular monitoring is important. Prevention and a combination of medication and lifestyle intervention have proven to obliterate or slow down the maternal and neonatal effects or complications of diabetes in pregnancy. During antenatal care in pregnancy; regular clinical checks on glycaemic control and other associated morbidities such as hypertension, preventive measures including dietary counselling, physical activity for adequate weight control, early identification of risk for complications from diabetes and constant communication with the pregnant woman on her current health state and the foetus are important [21, 23].

In most cases, the therapeutic management of GDM is with insulin therapy as oral hypoglycemic agents have not been proven to be safe due to concerns about potential teratogenicity and transport of glucose across the placenta [24, 25].

### 3.1 Monitoring

- Maternal metabolic surveillance should be directed at detecting hyperglycaemia severe enough to increase risks to the foetus. Daily self-monitoring of blood glucose (SMBG) appears superior to intermittent office monitoring of plasma glucose [26]. However, this will be initiated for those with a high risk of GDM or those already diagnosed with GDM.

- Glucose is found in the urine of over half of pregnant women, as such routine urine glucose checks may not be useful in GDM [27]. Any positive urine test result should be followed up with a blood glucose test.

- For women treated with insulin, limited evidence indicates that postprandial monitoring is superior to pre-prandial monitoring [28]. However, the success of either approach depends on the glycaemic targets that are set and achieved.

- Maternal surveillance should include blood pressure and urine protein monitoring to detect hypertensive disorders.

- Increased surveillance for pregnancies at risk for foetal demise is appropriate.

- The initiation, frequency, and specific techniques used to assess foetal well-being will depend on the cumulative risk the foetus bears from GDM and any other medical/obstetric conditions present.

- Early assessment for asymmetric foetal growth by ultrasonography, may aid in identifying foetuses that can benefit from maternal insulin therapy [29].

Likewise, for curative measures and at delivery, strict glycaemic surveillance and control with appropriate medications, monitored labour management and are the keystone of perinatal care for expectant mothers with diabetes, while new treatments/remedies for/that would benefit mother and child and prevent effects or complication of this state are continuously being worked on in the clinical and social settings [20].

### 3.2 Recommendations

In line with a globally or regionally accepted management for diabetes in pregnancy—a multidisciplinary team approach, multilevel healthcare system/setting, local policies and standardised clinical practice guidelines should be made available for continuation of care for both mother and child, especially in the postpartum period, to reduce the effect and complications of diabetes in pregnancy.

This is important because most available guidelines are made for the advanced or global north setting, majorly excluding point-of-contact care guidelines (asides from screening and referral) for basic primary or community-based healthcare centres, where most pregnant women first present or have their deliveries in the developing or global south countries. Likewise, more research work needs to be carried out on the social determinants of DM outcomes in mothers and babies, as it pertains to different localities and socio-economic classes across the globe.

## 4. Conclusion

GDM and PDM are important complications which can affect the pregnancy of different women. To ensure the appropriate management and delivery of a healthy child by a healthy mother, it is important to adequately screen high-risk mothers and implements the appropriate management strategies per guidelines.

## Acknowledgements

The authors would like to thank the academic society that has done extensive work on investigating diabetes in pregnancy.

## Conflict of interest

The authors declare no conflicts of interest.

*DOI: http://dx.doi.org/10.5772/intechopen.108564*

## Author details

Olakunmi Ololade Ogunyemi[1]*, Oluwakemi Mary Agoyi-Awoniyi[2] and Hassan Taiwo Yahaya[3]

1 OnTime Consortium, Nigeria

2 Safer Hands Initiative, Nigeria

3 Medical News Today, Nigeria

*Address all correspondence to: yemikunmi.o@gmail.com

IntechOpen

## References

[1] Chaya G, Eric K. Chapter 13—Diabetes mellitus. In: Chaya G, Erik K, editors. Biology of Cardiovascular and Metabolic Diseases. Academic Press; 2022. pp. 223-243

[2] Wilmot EG, Mansell P. Diabetes and pregnancy. Clinical Medicine. 2014;**14**(6):80. Available from: /pmc/articles/PMC4954145/

[3] Association AD. Gestational diabetes mellitus. Diabetes Care. 2003;**26**(suppl_1):s103-s105. Available from: https://diabetesjournals.org/care/article/26/suppl_1/s103/21729/Gestational-Diabetes-Mellitus

[4] Metzger BE, Lowe LP, Dyer AR, Chaovarindr U, Hospital R, Coustan DR, et al. Hyperglycaemia and adverse pregnancy outcomes. New England Journal of Medicine. 2008;**358**(19):1991-2002. Available from: https://www.nejm.org/doi/full/10.1056/NEJMoa0707943

[5] Chowdhury SR, Kamal AHM, Barua S, Ullah SMA. (PDF) The management of pre-existing diabetes in pregnancy : A review for primary care. Journal of Army Medical College Jashore. 2020;**1**(1):21-31. Available from: https://www.researchgate.net/publication/338828819_The_Management_of_Pre-Existing_Diabetes_in_Pregnancy_A_Review_for_Primary_Care

[6] Muche AA, Olayemi OO, Gete YK. Prevalence and determinants of gestational diabetes mellitus in Africa based on the updated international diagnostic criteria: A systematic review and meta-analysis. Archives of Public Health. 2019;**77**(1):1-20. Available from: https://archpublichealth.biomedcentral.com/articles/10.1186/s13690-019-0362-0

[7] Koo BK, Lee JH, Kim J, Jang EJ, Lee CH. Prevalence of gestational diabetes mellitus in korea: A national health insurance database study. PLoS One. 2016;**11**(4):e0153107. Available from: https://journals.plos.org/plosone/article?id=10.1371/journal.pone.0153107

[8] Melchior H, Kurch-Bek D, Mund M. The prevalence of gestational diabetes: A population-based analysis of a nationwide screening program. Deutsches Ärzteblatt International. 2017;**114**(24):412. Available from: /pmc/articles/PMC5499505/

[9] Lockitch G. Clinical biochemistry of pregnancy. Critical Reviews in Clinical Laboratory Sciences. 1997;**34**(1):67-139. Available from: https://pubmed.ncbi.nlm.nih.gov/9055057/

[10] Soma-Pillay P, Nelson-Piercy C, Tolppanen H, Mebazaa A. Physiological changes in pregnancy. Cardiovascular Journal of Africa. 2016;**27**(2):89. Available from:/pmc/articles/PMC4928162/

[11] Rodger M, Sheppard D, Gándara E, Tinmouth A. Haematological problems in obstetrics. Best Practice & Research. Clinical Obstetrics & Gynaecology. 2015;**29**(5):671-684. Available from:https://pubmed.ncbi.nlm.nih.gov/25819750/

[12] Wilson M, Morganti AA, Zervoudakis I, Letcher RL, Romney BM, von Oeyon P, et al. Blood pressure, the renin-aldosterone system and sex steroids throughout normal pregnancy. The American Journal of Medicine. 1980;**68**(1):97-104. Available from: https://pubmed.ncbi.nlm.nih.gov/7350810/

[13] Mean Fasting Blood Glucose . Available from: https://www.who.int/

data/gho/indicator-metadata-registry/imr-details/2380

[14] Dhillon KK, Gupta S. Biochemistry, Ketogenesis. StatPearls. 2022. Available from: https://www.ncbi.nlm.nih.gov/books/NBK493179/

[15] Yang HX. Diagnostic criteria for gestational diabetes mellitus (WS 331-2011). Chinese Medical Journal. 2012;**125**(7):1212-1213. Available from: https://journals.lww.com/cmj/Fulltext/2012/04010/Diagnostic_criteria_for_gestational_diabetes.4.aspx

[16] Moore TR. Diabetes Mellitus and Pregnancy 2022 . Available from: https://emedicine.medscape.com/article/127547-overview

[17] O'Sullivan JB. Establishing criteria for gestational diabetes. Diabetes Care. 1980;**3**(3):437-439. Available from: https://pubmed.ncbi.nlm.nih.gov/7389559/

[18] Ornoy A, Reece EA, Pavlinkova G, Kappen C, Miller RK. Effect of maternal diabetes on the embryo, foetus, and children: Congenital anomalies, genetic and epigenetic changes and developmental outcomes. Birth Defects Research. Part C, Embryo Today. 2015;**105**(1):53-72. Available from: https://onlinelibrary.wiley.com/doi/full/10.1002/bdrc.21090

[19] Muche AA, Olayemi OO, Gete YK. Effects of gestational diabetes mellitus on risk of adverse maternal outcomes: A prospective cohort study in Northwest Ethiopia. BMC Pregnancy and Childbirth. 2020;**20**(1):1-13. Available from: https://bmcpregnancychildbirth.biomedcentral.com/articles/10.1186/s12884-020-2759-8

[20] Zhuang W, Lv J, Liang Q, Chen W, Zhang S, Sun X. Adverse effects of gestational diabetes-related risk factors on pregnancy outcomes and intervention measures. Experimental and Therapeutic Medicine. 2020;**20**(4):3361. Available from: /pmc/articles/PMC7444321/

[21] Mitanchez D. Foetal and neonatal complications in gestational diabetes: perinatal mortality, congenital malformations, macrosomia, shoulder dystocia, birth injuries, neonatal complications. Diabetes & Metabolism. 2010;**36**(6 Pt 2):617-627. Available from: https://pubmed.ncbi.nlm.nih.gov/21163425/

[22] Narchi H, Kulaylat N. Heart disease in infants of diabetic mothers. Images in Paediatric Cardiology. 2000;**2**(2):17. Available from:/pmc/articles/PMC3232483/

[23] Daley B, Hitman G, Fenton N, Mclachlan S. Assessment of the methodological quality of local clinical practice guidelines on the identification and management of gestational diabetes. BMJ Open. 2019;**9**(6):e027285. Available from: https://bmjopen.bmj.com/content/9/6/e027285

[24] Muhwava LS, Murphy K, Zarowsky C, Levitt N. Policies and clinical practices relating to the management of gestational diabetes mellitus in the public health sector, South Africa - A qualitative study. BMC Health Services Research. 2018;**18**(1):1-16. Available from: https://bmchealthservres.biomedcentral.com/articles/10.1186/s12913-018-3175-x

[25] Turok DK, Ratcliffe SD, Baxley EG. Management of gestational diabetes mellitus. American Family Physician. 2003;**68**(9):1767-1773

[26] Kirk JK, Stegner J. Self-monitoring of blood glucose: Practical aspects. Journal of Diabetes Science and

Technology. 2010;**4**(2):435-439. DOI: 10.1177/193229681000400225

[27] Alto WA. No need for glycosuria/proteinuria screen in pregnant women. The Journal of Family Practice. 2005;**54**(11):978-983

[28] de Veciana M, Major CA, Morgan MA, Asrat T, Toohey JS, Lien JM, et al. Postprandial versus preprandial blood glucose monitoring in women with gestational diabetes mellitus requiring insulin therapy. The New England Journal of Medicine. 1995;**333**(19):1237-1241. DOI: 10.1056/NEJM199511093331901

[29] Brand JS, West J, Tuffnell D, et al. Gestational diabetes and ultrasound-assessed fetal growth in South Asian and White European women: Findings from a prospective pregnancy cohort. BMC Medicine. 2018;**16**:203. DOI: 10.1186/s12916-018-1191-7

Chapter 10

# Preterm Birth and Postnatal Developmental Outcomes

*Jamila Gurbanova, Saadat Huseynova and Afat Hasanova*


## Abstract

Premature birth is a pathological condition that requires high-quality medical care due to the infants' low body mass and gestational age, as well as morpho-functional immaturity. Moreover, such children are at great risk for retardation of mental development; metabolic, cardiovascular, and malignant diseases; and many other health problems at a later age. Early and late complications of preterm birth depend significantly on the gestational age at birth and the intrauterine development conditions of the fetus. Due to the more severe and complicated course of perinatal pathologies, premature babies with fetal growth retardation syndrome constitute a larger risk group. Approximately 50–70% of these children receive long-term treatment in the neonatal intensive care unit after birth. Furthermore, 70% of them face behavioral and memory problems in later life. While the pathologies of the neonatal period in children born prematurely are mainly related to respiratory, gastrointestinal, neurological, and nutritional problems, the complications of premature birth are manifested in children's early age, preschool, school, adolescence, and other developmental periods.


**Keywords:** preterm birth, neurodevelopmental disorders, perinatal encephalopathy, brain injury, perinatal prognostic indicators

## 1. Introduction

Premature birth is a pathological condition that requires high-quality medical care due to the infants' low body mass and gestational age, as well as morphofunctional immaturity. Moreover, such children are at great risk for retardation of mental development; metabolic, cardiovascular, and malignant diseases; and many other health problems at a later age [1, 2]. Early and late complications of preterm birth depend significantly on the gestational age at birth and the intrauterine development conditions of the fetus [3, 4]. Due to the more severe and complicated course of perinatal pathologies, premature babies with fetal growth retardation syndrome constitute a larger risk group. Approximately 50–70% of these children receive long-term treatment in the neonatal intensive care unit after birth. Furthermore, 70% of them face behavioral and memory problems in later life [5, 6].

Children with extreme small mass comprise a significant risk group due to developmental and behavioral anomalies. The main problems faced by these children in the neonatal period are related to nutrition and infection [7]. Thus, not only satisfying the energy demand, but also the oral and parenteral intake of the necessary nutrients and microelements leads to the prevention of a number of psychosocial problems at later ages [8, 9]. Additionally, the correct use of antibiotics, the timely implementation of measures to protect against hospital bacterial strains, and the minimization of damage to the integrity of the skin and mucous membranes lead to the reduction of infectious complications [10, 11]. One of the factors leading to the violation of early adaptation in children born prematurely is the immaturity of the painful stimuli response. It is believed that because gestational age and the degree of morphofunctional maturity of the body are low, the cumulative reaction formed in the body against pain stimulus causes not only behavioral disorders but also dysfunctional changes in all organs and systems [12, 13].

Premature birth is the most important medical and social problem of modern times, accounting for 12% of all live births [14]. The rate of prematurity in child mortality varies according to the level of neonatal care in a given region [15]. According to the Institute of Children's Health and Development, this problem ranks first among causes of child mortality in the African-American zone and second in the Caucasian zone [15, 16]. Despite the improvement of preventive and treatment measures in this field, the fact that the frequency of premature birth is increasing all over the world can be explained by the low level of neonatal care in some regions and the increase in the number of multi-fetal pregnancies as a result of the widespread use of assisted reproductive technologies in developed countries [17, 18]. Statistical studies have shown that even in developed countries, pregnancy ending with premature birth has increased from 9 to 9.4% to 12.7–14% compared to the 1980s [1, 19]. An estimated 75% of the 500,000 preterm births that occur worldwide each year are between 34 and 36 weeks of gestational age, with 25% at a lower gestational age [20–22]. Studies have shown that 50% of all preterm births occur spontaneously without any specific cause, 40% are medically induced, and 10% occur due to the premature rupture of fetal membranes [23].

Among the risk factors leading to premature birth, in recent years, a history of complicated incomplete birth, multiple pregnancy, and short cervical length have become increasingly relevant. It is believed that women whose previous pregnancies ended prematurely have a higher risk of stillbirth. The recurrent risk depends on the gestational age of the child born during the previous pregnancy and the number of premature births in the history of the woman. Thus, in 50–70% of cases, incomplete birth is repeated at the same gestational age. As well, the risk of repeated preterm birth is 16% in women who have given birth to one child at a gestational age of less than 35 weeks and 41–67% in women who have had multiple pregnancies [24, 25]. Due to the widespread use of assisted reproductive technologies, the number of multiple pregnancies has increased significantly in the last 20 years. Although in vitro fertilization is more successful at achieving and sustaining pregnancy, most twin and multiple pregnancies result in preterm birth [26, 27]. A number of studies have confirmed the association of short cervix size with preterm birth. Some authors have even proposed predicting the time of childbirth based on this indicator [28, 29]. Randomized clinical trials have shown that vaginal progesterone treatment to reduce the risk of premature termination of pregnancy with short cervical length had a positive effect in 45% of cases [25, 30].

Investigations into the possible causes of spontaneous births have found that the intrauterine inflammatory process, mother's psychosocial stress, fetal psychological stress, uterine overstretching, and uterine bleeding are of significant note [31–34]. These causes manifest themselves with different frequency depending on the duration of pregnancy. For example, births stimulated by intrauterine bacterial colonization usually occur at a gestational age of less than 34 weeks, while pregnancies that end due to psychosocial problems occur at a gestational age of 34–36 weeks. Preeclampsia, fetal distress, and retardation of fetal development are the main pregnancy pathologies that cause premature birth. According to the data of the International Institute for Child Health and Development, 40% of premature births due to medical intervention are related to women with preeclampsia [35–37]. Premature rupture of fetal membranes occurs mainly as a result of exacerbation of chronic inflammation, accounting for 21% and 8% of early and late preterm births, respectively [38]. Studies have shown that placental inflammation caused by the impaired protective capacity of the antioxidant protein heme oxygenase-1 plays a fundamental role in the pathogenesis of both preeclampsia and the premature rupture of fetal membranes. Therefore, some scientific studies have been conducted on the effectiveness of drugs with heme oxygenase activity to prolong pregnancy when there is a risk of premature birth [39, 40]. Parturition is a complex biological process regulated by numerous signaling molecules and biologically active substances from the mother, mate, and fetal tissue. A number of preventive measures are implemented to identify and prevent the risk of premature birth. Studies have shown that the placental corticotropin-releasing hormone is the main endocrine mediator of preterm labor [41, 42]. Determination of this factor in pregnancies with a gestation period of less than 33 weeks can be a prognostic indicator of the level of fetal development and premature birth [43–45]. In recent years, the use of special portable monitors that monitor children's activity at home has been proposed, but this method is not widely used due to the high economic costs required. The dynamic monitoring of women to prevent any problems that may occur during pregnancy, tocolytic therapy to reduce uterine contractions if necessary, and antibiotic therapy in case of infectious complications are believed to be more effective. Of course, since women whose previous pregnancies ended in premature birth are at greater risk, they should be monitored more actively. The most successful results in the prevention of recurrent premature births have been obtained via the administration of 12 alpha-hydroxyprogesterone injections. Thus, prescribing this drug to women whose previous pregnancies ended in premature birth at 16–20 weeks of gestation significantly reduces the risk of premature birth [46–48].

Fetal inflammatory response is the main pathogenetic link to preterm birth. The process is due to the influence of microorganisms and is accompanied by chorioamnionitis, funisitis, or intraamnial inflammation [49, 50]. Acute intraventricular hemorrhage, periventricular leukomalacia (PVL), necrotic enterocolitis, bronchopulmonary dysplasia, myocardial dysfunction, and sepsis are more common during the inflammatory process of the fetoplacental system [51–54]. During the fetal inflammatory response, preterm birth is associated with the effects of cytokines, matrix metalloproteinases, and prostaglandins. In cases of high bacterial colonization, the levels of TNF-$\alpha$, IL-6, and IL-8 in umbilical cord blood increase significantly [55, 56]. The main clinical manifestations of inflammatory changes that lead to premature birth are uterine prolapse, changes in the cervix, and the premature rupture of the fetal membranes. Unfortunately, during the inflammatory process occurring in the fetoplacental system, the risk of similar inflammation in the mother's body is very low. Therefore, it is not possible to predict preterm birth based on the inflammatory indicators in the peripheral blood of pregnant women. The cultivation of microbial colonization determined during the examination of the contents taken from the birth canal also does not provide an idea of the level of intraamniotic inflammation [32, 57, 58]. The decrease in the probability of premature birth against the background of antibiotic therapy is also explained by the inhibition of the bacterial infectious process due to the effect of antibacterial drugs [59]. However, there are conflicting and controversial opinions on the use of antibiotic therapy to reduce the probability of premature termination of pregnancy [60–62]. A group of studies has shown that routine treatment of asymptomatic microbial invasion reduces perinatal morbidity and mortality but has no effect on the incidence of preterm birth [63–65]. Other studies have shown that bacterial colonization increases the risk of premature birth, although it is not manifested by a specific infectious process. In cervical and vaginal secretions, a membrane protein called fetal fibronectin is found at a frequency 50 times higher in women with the possibility of premature birth than in those with normal pregnancies [66, 67]. The Maternal-Fetal Medicine Union states that the reduction of fetal fibronectin does not occur against the background of antibiotic therapy [68–70]. As well, despite the weakening of intrauterine colonization against the background of antibacterial therapy, against the background of the use of broad-spectrum antibiotics, no significant improvement in spontaneous births or perinatal and neonatal outcomes has been shown [62, 70]. Therefore, for more accurate diagnosis and data, the contents obtained directly from the fetal membranes rather than from the birth canal should be examined. Elevation of IL-6 and matrix metalloproteinase 8 and 9 levels in amniotic fluid is also considered a more sensitive indicator for amniotic infection [71, 72]. However, because obtaining amniotic fluid is invasive and poses a risk for subsequent infection, this diagnostic method is not widely used. In recent years, it has been considered more appropriate to differentiate inflammatory processes in the amniotic cavity, chorion, and placenta through vaginal cervicometry [73, 74]. Thus, when intraamniotic microbial colonization increases, in 80% of cases, the length of the cervix is shortened, which is called cervical insufficiency [75–77]. This method is safer and is now widely used in predicting the occurrence of premature birth. Another group of studies has shown that fetal damage during microbial colonization depends on the activity of anti-inflammatory factors in the fetoplacental system. It was determined that as a result of the effect of oxidative stress products, the activation of specific soluble and transmembrane RAGE receptors occurs in macrophages, monocytes, and endothelial cells [78]. This directly leads to the activation of cytokine and growth factor genes [79, 80]. The activation of RAGE receptors during the acceleration of the inflammatory process have been proven to have a protective nature, causing the inhibition of inflammation [81]. Another group of studies has shown that the progress and activity of the inflammatory process depends on the degree of activation of the RAGE and Toll-like receptors [82, 83]. Taketoshi Noguchi and co-authors showed that activation of Toll-like receptors induces preterm labor by leading to a more acute inflammatory process in the fetoplacental system [84]. The activation of RAGE receptors causes the inhibition of the acute process, and the process becomes chronic [85, 86]. A group of studies proved that the polymorphism of Toll-like receptors and the genetic structure of different alleles play an important role in the occurrence of premature birth [87, 88]. Hopefully, large-scale scientific research is being conducted on the genetic basis of the occurrence of premature birth. According to the obtained results thus far, premature pregnancy depends on cytokine, Toll-like receptors, and RAGE polymorphism regulated at the genetic level. Depending on this polymorphism, the inflammatory response of the fetoplacental system is formed. This response, in turn, not only causes premature birth but also significantly affects the course of perinatal pathologies [89]. Uteroplacental ischemia is primarily formed during the inflammatory process in the mother-couple-fetus system [89, 90]. At this time, generalized endothelial dysfunction leads to premature termination of pregnancy and various intrauterine developmental pathologies of the fetus [91]. The pathogenetic mechanisms of the formation of endothelial dysfunction during uteroplacental ischemia have not yet been fully investigated. However, numerous scientific studies have proven that inflammatory processes occurring in the fetoplacental system are often accompanied by thrombophilic conditions [1, 92, 93]. Thrombophilia factors that lead to premature birth are grouped into two categories—congenital and acquired. Congenital thrombophilia is mainly caused by the Leiden mutation and coagulation factor II - prothrombin mutation [94]. Antiphospholipid syndrome is the main acquired factor [95]. The violation of placental microcirculation during thrombophilia can cause thromboembolism, intrauterine death of the fetus, intrauterine growth retardation, premature separation of the pair, acute preeclampsia, and spontaneous abortions [52, 96, 97].

In recent scientific literature, there have been many reports on the increased incidence of preterm birth in women with mutations of the methylenetetrahydrofolate reductase gene and disorders of folic acid metabolism [98]. It is believed that as a result of mutation, folic acid cannot be activated and transformed into tetrahydrafolate-metafolin. As the latter provides the remethylation of homocysteine, its deficiency leads to disruption of homocysteine transformation and its excessive accumulation in the body [99]. Hyperhomocysteinemia causes generalized damage to the endothelium, atherosclerotic changes, placental microcirculation disorders, premature birth, sudden intrauterine death, as well as congenital developmental anomalies of the neural tube, heart, and a number of organs [100–102].

One of the main reasons for premature termination of pregnancy is the improper adjustment of the contraction capacity of the uterine muscle depending on the period of gestation. Contraction of the uterus is regulated by the interaction of actin and myosin proteins in myocytes [103]. Myocytes, which create special connections, ensure the synchrony and coordination of contractions of the uterus. The interaction of the actin and myosin complex is realized by the phosphorylation of myosin by the enzyme myosinkinase. The homeostasis of calcium ions plays a key role in myocyte activity. The increase in calcium ions inside the cell is carried out through membrane receptors stimulated by ovarian and placental steroids. Progesterone activates beta adrenergic receptors, and estradiol activates alpha adrenergic, cholinergic, and prostaglandin receptors [104, 105]. The passage of calcium ions into the cell membrane is carried out by alpha adrenergic receptor agonists, and its return is carried out by beta adrenergic receptor agonists. The contraction and relaxation of the uterine muscle depends on the entry of calcium ions from the sarcoplasmic reticulum into the cytoplasm and the amount of agonists and antagonists of multiple receptors involved in this process [106, 107]. Depending on their balance, inadequate contraction of the uterine muscle, loss of synchrony prompts the onset of premature labor. It has been established that uterine contractions during childbirth and labor pains are initiated through the expression of contraction-related protein genes [108, 109]. These genes regulate the synthesis of Connexin-43, the main protein of ion channels and receptors [110]. The role of a number of factors in the regulation of the synchrony of uterine contractions has been indicated—notably, progesterone, nitric oxide, relaxin, prostacyclin, and the corticotropin-releasing hormone (CRH) [110–112]. These biologically active substances, called hestagens, prevent the release of calcium ions from the sarcoplasmic reticulum by inhibiting cyclic AMF inside the cell. Since numerous experimental studies have shown that these compounds reduce inadequate uterine contractions, they are now widely used in clinical practice to prevent premature birth.

There are many theories about the immunological incompatibility between the mother and the fetus in the etiopathogenesis of premature birth. Increased tolerance of the mother to the fetus depends on the balance of the histological compatibility of complex antigens. While class I HLA-A and HLA-B antigens can be inactivated by the trophoblast, HLA-G antigens expressed during pregnancy protect the fetus from the maternal immune response [102, 113]. Inadequate recognition of fetal antigens by the mother can lead to miscarriage. In animal studies, reduction of galectin-1, a specific immunoregulatory protein, has been shown to stimulate preterm labor [114]. Additionally, in the case of a number of autoimmune diseases (systemic lupus erythematosus, ulcerative colitis, immunopathologies of the thyroid gland, etc.), there is a high probability of premature birth, and the severity of immunological incompatibility between the mother and the fetus significantly affects the gestation period at which the birth ends [106, 115]. In a number of studies, opinions have been expressed about the allergic reaction of the mother to fetal tissues during pregnancy [116, 117]. According to relevant sources, the amount of eosinophilic granulocytes in the amniotic fluid increases in cases of premature birth. As well, the number of mast cells, more sensitive to allergic processes, is greater in the uterine muscle, and due to the effect of prostaglandin, they easily degranulate and accelerate the accumulation of the uterus. Currently, scientific studies are being conducted to study the effectiveness of antihistamine drugs in preventing premature birth [118].

Congenital anomalies of the uterus, polyhydramnios, and the high risk of premature birth during multiple pregnancy indicate that uterine muscle tension plays an important role in pregnancy disruption. Although the size of the uterus increases as the pregnancy period increases, the intrauterine tension remains constant. Progesterone and endogenous myometrial relaxants, especially nitric oxide, are important in maintaining this stability [119, 120]. Prostaglandins and neuromuscular junction proteins, especially connexin-43, increase during uterine strain [121]. Amniochorial strain, on the other hand, causes the premature rupture of membranes and premature birth. Because of this, premature birth is more difficult to control and is regarded as an almost unavoidable process.

Thus, although numerous concepts of the causes and pathophysiology of premature birth have been put forward and various developmental mechanisms have been determined, it is not possible to completely prevent perinatal pathologies caused by premature termination of pregnancy or incomplete birth. Although inflammation has been identified as the main pathogenetic mechanism in the occurrence of premature birth, the pathophysiology of the process has not yet been fully studied. The inflammatory process in the fetoplacental system is stimulated both by the effect of bacterial colonization and by the effect of hypoxia, accompanied by an inflammatory response in the maternal and fetal bodies. However, since the response to fetal infection is often not manifested by noticeable pathological changes in a pregnant woman, it can be overlooked by specialists or identified late. Even if it does not cause a pathological process in the mother's body, the fetal inflammatory response causes premature birth, increased perinatal morbidity, and mortality. In modern times, despite the improvement of perinatal medical care technologies, methods for the effective prevention of premature birth have not been developed. The specificity and sensitivity of clinical-instrumental examinations and laboratory markers are very low. Therefore, in recent years, numerous scientific studies have been conducted with the aim of finding new sensitive markers of premature birth and identifying women from the risk group by involving pregnant women in screening examinations.

## 2. Preterm birth and perinatal prognostic indicators of further age pathologies

Due to the high level of technology and quality medical care in the field of neonatology in recent years, noticeable achievements have been made in reducing the mortality rates of small and extremely small premature babies [100, 122]. In many countries, the criteria for live birth have been changed and great achievements have been made in feeding children whose gestational age is older than 22 weeks [123–125]. Although the number of survivors among children born at 23–24 weeks of gestational age has increased, a number of early and late complications among them have become a serious medical and social problem. While the pathologies of the neonatal period in children born prematurely are mainly related to respiratory, gastrointestinal, neurological, and nutritional problems, the complications of premature birth are manifested in children's early age, preschool, school, adolescence, and other developmental periods [126–128].

The lower the gestational age, the more severe are the long-term consequences of a preterm birth. Even in profoundly premature babies without structural changes in the brain, minimal brain dysfunctions are manifested in further development. Deeply premature babies, whose neonatal period is complicated by various pathologies, always require long-term monitoring and rehabilitation [129, 130]. After discharge from neonatal intensive care units, neuro-developmental abnormalities are the most common problem for premature babies. The most common neurodevelopmental anomalies include cerebral palsy, various forms of psychomotor development and behavioral disorders, as well as vision and hearing problems [131–135].

The timely detection of neurodevelopmental delays and implementation of rehabilitation measures lead to a significant reduction in the severity and complications of later age problems. Therefore, in a number of developed countries, monitoring the development of premature children is carried out at the state level, and multicenter randomized clinical studies are given great importance. The lower the age of gestation and the degree of morphofunctional maturity of the brain, the more common are secondary brain damage in hypoxia-ischemia, sepsis, necrotic enterocolitis, meningitis and other infectious inflammatory processes; nutritional disorders are more common in these children, which manifests itself in various ways at later ages. It shows with developmental problems of degree [136–139]. In particular, organic damage to the brain—intraventricular hemorrhage, periventricular leukomalacia, and gross psychomotor developmental disorders with ventriculomegaly, including infantile cerebral palsy, are more likely [140, 141].

Radiological examinations have important diagnostic value in the acute period of brain damage and can form certain ideas about future neurodevelopmental problems [122, 142]. However, at present, the results of early ultrasound examinations are hardly used as a prognostic indicator of neuromotor development. According to the studies by Laptook and co-authors, the specificity and sensitivity of abnormal neurosonography results are very low; cerebral palsy is noted in 9.4% of children with a body mass of less than 1000 g and a normal brain ultrasound examination [143, 144]. In the last few decades, the topical diagnosis of brain injuries has started to be performed using magnetic resonance imaging (MRI), and successful results have been achieved in this direction. While significant changes in brain white matter during the acute phase of central nervous system injuries are detected by ultrasound, MRI is a more sensitive imaging modality for identifying smaller brain lesions [145–147]. Cerebellar lesions, which are difficult to detect by ultrasound, can also be successfully diagnosed by MRI [148]. As a result of this MRI use, monitoring the subsequent development of children with various changes in the brain has led to the discovery of valuable prognostic information [149]. The positive and negative prognostic value of the changes determined as a result of the examination varies depending on the severity of the damage, the gestational age of the child, and the influence of environmental factors affecting developmental delay. For example, among children with white matter damage at the age of five, while the negative prognostic value of a normal MRI for neurodevelopmental retardation is 100%, the positive prognostic value is 75%, excluding cognitive impairment [150–152].

Considering the presence of numerous factors that can affect cognitive development in later development, it can be considered legitimate that there is no relationship between perinatal white matter damage and cognitive development disorders. Studies have shown that diffuse white matter damage causes neuromotor retardation in preschool and school-aged children [153, 154]. In the research done at Turku University in Finland, it was noted that in premature babies, this examination is carried out not only in the first days after birth but also at the age equivalent to term birth, which leads to the acquisition of honest prognostic information about the development of neuromotor functions in the first five years of life. The essence of this scientific conclusion is that the changes detected as a result of MRI only in adult brain tissue cause neurodevelopmental disorders at later ages [155]. It is believed that the development of the brain mass is proportional to the growth of the head circumference, and the child's neuro-motor development can be evaluated and predicted based on this indicator. As a result of MRI examination, it is possible to determine the total volume of the brain, and in children born with a very small mass, the volume of the total or individual parts of the brain has a significant impact on the mental, speech, memory, and psychomotor indicators of the child's further development [156]. Structural damage detected during MRI examination is not always equivalent to brain dysfunction. Thus, psychomotor development may be completely normal in cases where noticeable pathologies are detected [157]. However, in all cases, MRI examination surpasses many development scales and immunohistochemical markers determined on the basis of clinical indicators according to its prognostic value.

Studies on the assessment of early neurological development in premature infants have shown that cerebral palsy and behavioral-developmental pathologies are of greater relevance. Such pathologies are accompanied by abnormal muscle tone and movement disorders, and the clinical course and prognosis depend on the direction in which the motor functions change. Thus, more functional and sensory disorders are observed in hemiplegia and diplegia, while more motor disorders are found in triplegia and quadriplegia [158].

Cerebral palsy is distinguished according to the degree of severity as follows: mild (the child has only mild movement disorders, general muscle activity does not lag behind age norms), moderate (the child can walk with assistive devices, can sit freely), and severe (the child has the ability to move, no assistive devices can be activated) [159]. Of course, along the course of the pathological process, a number of external interventions and the prescription of drugs significantly affect the prognostic indicators. For example, the administration of antenatal steroids and indomethacin in the perinatal period reduces the risk of intraventricular hemorrhage [160]. Corticosteroids used postnatally in the treatment and prevention of bronchopulmonary dysplasia in premature infants increase the risk of developing cerebral palsy [161–163]. In general, according to the incidence of psychomotor developmental pathologies of early age, those born with deep prematurity and extreme small mass are at greater risk, with such pathologies occurring in 9–17% of children who survive various perinatal pathologies [164, 165]. Numerous scientific research projects have been carried out on the further development of children born prematurely; over time, the results found through this research have differed fundamentally from one study to another. Information about classical randomized studies entered the periodical literature in the 1970s. If the first epidemiological studies were devoted only to the study of the form and frequency of developmental delays, since the 1990s, the effectiveness of various scales and diagnostic markers to assess psychomotor and sensory development became the objects of research. Within the framework of the International Institute on Child Health and Development, the assessment of children aged 18–22 months after birth began for the first time, using the Classification System of Gross Motor Development, the Bailey Scale of Children's Development Assessment, and the Amiel–Thison scale of neurological development [92, 150].

In the twentieth century, starting from the perinatal period, various assessment and development programs were implemented one after the other, and large-scale scientific research was carried out in the search for more sensitive indicators of various neuromotor disorders. At present, the Bailey-2 scale of developmental assessment, Denver developmental screening test, CAT/CLAMS scale, and Gessel and Mullen comprehension tests are widely used [134, 166, 167]. The Denver screening test and its modified variants detect and predict gross motor, fine motor, social adaptation, and speech problems in the first 6 years of life starting from the first months after birth [168, 169]. Evaluation by this scale is currently considered the ideal test system for identifying children with developmental delays, playing the role of screening. Evaluation with the Beley scale and its modified versions allows for the detection of the severity of the pathological process in several ways and various clinical forms in children with developmental delays detected through screening [170, 171].

Developmental assessment tests are used to identify and predict the retardation of children's mental and psychomotor development levels in each developmental period. Based on the obtained results, timely preventive measures can lead to the prevention of a number of developmental delays. However, assessment and prediction based on these scales have several difficulties. Specifically, the accuracy of predictions is influenced by a number of external factors, including the social environment surrounding the child, educational level of the parents, and structural changes of the brain with various origins. Furthermore, it is not always possible to involve parents and children in such assessments in a timely and regular manner given that examinations take a long time.

Cognitive and behavioral reactions are of great importance in the proper formation of children's social adaptation. Profoundly preterm infants and children with intrauterine growth retardation constitute a greater risk group for the formation of cognitive functions on a weak basis [127, 172]. It is believed that both the antenatal and postnatal retardation of the child lead to a delay in behavioral and cognitive functions [173]. The psychological state of parents has a significant impact on the behavioral problems of premature children. Studies have found that there is a statistically significant relationship between parents' stress index and children's behavioral responses at 3 years of age [174]. In another study, it was shown that depressive symptoms in mothers led to impaired social adaptation and behavioral responses of children aged 5 years [175]. Experts who study the impact of nutrition on development have sought to prove that the formation of cognitive reactions does not differ in children who lag behind in antenatal or postnatal development and depends more on proper and balanced nutrition [176, 177]. Many authors have confirmed that there is a dependence between a child's weight and height parameters at birth and physical, psychomotor, and neurological development at later ages. According to Tanabe K. and co-authors, 18.2% of children with intrauterine growth retardation are stunted at school age. In children born with prematurity and intrauterine growth retardation syndrome, various changes occur in the central nervous system, and many are maintained for a long time without recovery at a later age [39, 119]. Especially in deep premature babies, pathologies such as cerebral hemorrhage, periventricular leukomalacia, and hypertension-hydrocephalus syndrome cannot be fully recovered despite continuous dispensary control, proper intensive therapy, and rehabilitation treatment [87, 178]. P. Casolini created experimental subneurotoxic anoxia in mice in the first week of life and observed persistent dysfunction of the hippocampus and cerebral cortex as well as the disruption of behavioral responses in subsequent development [179]. In another scientific study, the results of magnetic resonance examinations showed that in children born with low weight, the development of various structures of the brain was not proportional—the amount of gray matter in some areas was low and was maintained for a long time [180]. The disproportionate development of brain structures in children born with low weight was accompanied by physical and sexual underdevelopment at different ages, disruption of social adaptation, and attention disorders [171, 181, 182].

Research conducted over many years has concluded that in addition to psychomotor developmental delays, somatic and infectious pathologies of various organs and systems are also more likely to occur in the further development of children born prematurely. Children born with low birth weight have a high risk of death due to cardiovascular pathology [1]. Epidemiological studies conducted jointly by several perinatal scientific centers have proven that intrauterine growth retardation created experimentally as a result of hypoxia and nutrient deficiency in pregnant mice was a major risk factor for the development of cardiovascular diseases in later development is a risk [166, 183, 184]. Left ventricular remodeling of the heart has proven that ultrastructural changes caused by both ischemia and nutrient deficiency lead to future cardiac dysfunction [1].

Research on the genetic basis of organ dysfunction has led to certain results. For example, in studies conducted on mice, the removal of the NR2B fraction from the C terminus of the NMDA receptor gene, which plays an important role in the pathogenesis of perinatal damage to the nervous system, resulted in perinatal death. Another group of researchers observed a substantial decrease in NR1 and NR2B subunits as a result of biochemical tests in mice whose mothers were stressed during pregnancy. Later, electrophysiological studies revealed that intrauterine stress causes memory and cognitive impairments in later life as a result of the long-term dysfunction of the hippocampus [179, 180].

Many diagnostic and preventive programs have been proposed to prevent near and far consequences of preterm birth [130, 185, 186]. A number of sources have suggested a control program for children born with intrauterine growth retardation in polyclinic conditions, which serves to reduce their morbidity [23]. Depending on the variant of intrauterine growth retardation syndrome, dynamic dispensary control leads to a decrease in morbidity in such children. G.K. Swamy, with his research, has shown that timely and correct perinatal care has the leading role in reducing the morbidity and mortality rates of premature babies at a later age [187]. However, he has noted that even state-of-the-art medical care does little to reduce perinatal and postnatal morbidity in children born with severe and extreme low birth weight.

## 3. Conclusion

Thus, since the mechanisms of the formation of perinatal-period pathologies in children born prematurely have not yet been fully studied, early and late prevention of most diseases associated with the period of intrauterine development is not possible. However, problems of intrauterine development lie in the genesis of many diseases that appear in later development. Endothelial function is the basis of the formation mechanisms of the immune response to the inflammatory process in the fetoplacental system. Not only in the intrauterine period, but also in the early adaptation period after birth, due to the influence of various exogenous and endogenous factors, changes in the vasoregulatory and inflammatory response of the vascular endothelium affect the manifestation of diseases that appear in later development to one degree or another. Given the nature of the relationship between the inflammatory markers of individual organs and systems and the indicators of endothelial dysfunction, it is not possible to determine the perinatal risk factors affecting the future development of the body, but a wide range of scientific research is being conducted in this direction. Investigating the influence of the level of perinatal organ and endothelial dysfunction markers on further development, as well as the regional characteristics of premature birth, can be the basis for creating a perinatal prevention program for early-age pathologies.

## Author details

Jamila Gurbanova, Saadat Huseynova* and Afat Hasanova
Scientific Research Institute of Obstetrics and Gynecology, Azerbaijan

*Address all correspondence to: sadi_0105@mail.ru

## References

[1] Gaillard R, Steegers E, Tiemeier H, Hofman A, Jaddoe V. Placental vascular dysfunction, fetal and childhood growth, and cardiovascular development. Circulation. 2013;**128**:2202-2210

[2] Liu L, Johnson HL, Cousens S, Perin J, Scott S, Lawn JE, et al. Global, regional, and national causes of child mortality: An updated systematic analysis for 2010 with time trends since 2000. Lancet. 2012;**379**:2151-2161

[3] Katz J, Lee AC, Kozuki N, Lawn JE, Cousens S, et al. Mortality risk in preterm and small-for-gestational-age infants in low-income and middle-income countries: A pooled country analysis. The Lancet. 2013;**382**:417-425

[4] Risnes KR, Vatten LJ, Baker JL, Jameson K, Sovio U, et al. Birthweight and mortality in adulthood: A systematic review and meta-analysis. International Journal of Epidemiology. 2011;**40**:647-661

[5] Simchen MJ, Beiner ME, Strauss-Liviathan N, Dulitzky M, Kuint J, et al. Neonatal outcome in growth-restricted versus appropriately grown preterm infants. American Journal of Perinatology. 2000;**17**:187-192

[6] Souza JP, Gulmezoglu AM, Vogel J, Carroli G, Lumbiganon P, et al. Moving beyond essential interventions for reduction of maternal mortality (the WHO Multicountry Survey on Maternal and Newborn Health): A cross-sectional study. Lancet. 2013;**381**:1747-1755

[7] Eric CE, Stark AR. Management and outcomes of very low birth weight. The New England Journal of Medicine. 2008;**358**(16):1701-1711

[8] Trindade CEP. Minerals in the nutrition of extremely low birth weight infants. Jornal de Pediatria. 2005;**81**(1(Suppl)):43-51

[9] Darlow BA, Cust AE, Donoghue DA. Improved outcomes for very low birth weight infants: Evidence from New Zealand national population based data. Archives of Disease in Childhood. Fetal and Neonatal Edition. 2003;**88**(1):F23-F28

[10] Koo WW, Hockman EM. Posthospital discharge feeding for preterm infants: Effects of standard compared with enriched milk formula on growth, bone mass, and body composition. American Journal of Clinical Nutrition. 2006;**84**:1357-1364

[11] Meinzen-Derr J et al. Role of human milk in extremely low birth weight infants' risk of necrotizing enterocolitis or death. Journal of Perinatology. 2009;**29**:57-62

[12] Carbajal R, Rousset A, Danan C, et al. Epidemiology and treatment of painful procedures in neonates in intensive care units. Journal of the American Medical Association. 2008;**300**(1):60-70

[13] Grunau RE, Haley DW, Whitfield MF, et al. Altered basal cortisol levels at 3, 6, 8 and 18 months in preterm infants born at extremely low gestational age. The Journal of Pediatrics. 2007;**150**:151-156

[14] Reddy UM, Ko CW, Raju TNK, Willinger M. Delivery indications at late-preterm gestations and infant mortality rates in the United States. Pediatrics. 2009;**124**:234-240

[15] Goldenberg RL, Culhane JF, Iams JD, Romero R. Epidemiology and

causes of preterm birth. The Lancet. 2008;**371**(9606):75-84

[16] Mathews TJ, MacDorman MF. Infant mortality statistics from the 2006 period linked birth/infant death data set. National Vital Statistics Reports. 2010;**58**(17):1-32

[17] Lucja B, Gold C. Early intervention for premature infants in neonatal intensive care unit. Acta Neuropsychologica. 2014;**12**(2):185-203

[18] Norman J, Greer I. Preterm Labour, Managing Risk in Clinical Practice. Cambridge: Cambridge University Press; 2011

[19] Wallace ME, Mendola P, Chen Z, Grantz KL. Preterm birth in the context of increasing income inequality. Maternal and Child Health Journal. 2016;**20**(1):164-171. DOI: 10.1007/s10995-015-1816-9

[20] Althabe F, Belizan JM, McClure EM, HemingwayFoday J, Berrueta M, Mazzoni A, et al. A population-based, multifaceted strategy to implement antenatal corticosteroid treatment versus standard care for the reduction of neonatal mortality due to preterm birth in low-income and middle-income countries: The ACT cluster-randomised trial. Lancet. 2015;**385**(9968):629-639

[21] Conde-Agudelo A, Diaz-Rossello JL. Kangaroo mother care to reduce morbidity and mortality in low birthweight infants. Cochrane Database of Systematic Reviews. 2014;**4**:CD002771

[22] Kinney MV, Lawn JE, Howson CP, Belizan J. 15 million preterm births annually: What has changed this year? Reproductive Health. 2012;**9**:28

[23] Black RE, Cousens S, Johnson HL, Lawn JE, Rudan I, Bassani DG, et al. Global, regional, and national causes of child mortality in 2008: A systematic analysis. Lancet. 2010;**375**(9730):1969-1987

[24] Wong L, Wilkes J, Korgenski K, Varner MW, Manuck TA. Risk factors associated with preterm birth after a prior term delivery. BJOG. 2016;**123**(11):1772-1778. DOI: 10.1111/1471-0528.13683

[25] Norwitz ER, Phaneuf LE, Caughey AB. Progesterone supplementation and the prevention of preterm birth. Reviews in Obstetrics and Gynecology. 2011;**4**(2):60-72

[26] McDonald SD, Han Z, Mulla S, Murphy KE, Beyene J, Ohlsson A. Preterm birth and low birth weight among in vitrofertilization singletons: A systematic review and meta-analyses. EJOG. 2009;**146**(2):138-148

[27] Wisborg K, Ingerslev HJ, Henriksen TB. In vitro fertilization and preterm delivery, low birth weight, and admission to the neonatal intensive care unit: A prospective follow-up study. Fertility and Sterility. 2010;**94**(6):2102-2106

[28] Lu L, Qu Y, Tang J, Chen D, Mu D. Risk factors associated with late preterm births in the underdeveloped region of China: A cohort study and systematic review. Taiwanese Journal of Obstetrics and Gynecology. 2015;**54**:647-653

[29] Barber MA, Eguiluz I, Plasencia W, Medina M, Valle L, Garcia JA. Preterm delivery and ultrasound measurement of cervical length in Gran Canaria, Spain. International Journal of Gynecology & Obstetrics. 2010;**108**:58-60

[30] Mesiano S, Wang X, Norwitz ER. Progesterone receptors in the human pregnancy uterus: Do they hold the key to birth timing? Reproductive Sciences. 2011;**18**:6-19

[31] Asuquo B, Vellone AD, Walters G, Manney S, Miquimi L, Kurst H. A case-control study of teh risk of adverse perinatal outcomes due to tuberculosis during pregnancy. Journal of Obstetrics and Gynaecology. 2012;**32**:635-638. DOI: 10.3109/01443615. 2012.704436

[32] George LM, Nadeem OK, Quinlivan JA. Bacterial aetiological agents of intra-amniotic infections and preterm birth in pregnant women. Frontiers in Cellular and Infection Microbiology. 2013;**3**:58-65

[33] Hobel CJ. Stress and preterm birth. Clinical Obstetrics and Gynecology. 2004;**47**(4):856-880

[34] McDonald SW, Kingston D, Bayrampour H, Dolan SM, Tough SC. Cumulative psychosocial stress, coping resources, and preterm birth. Archives of Women's Mental Health. 2014;**17**(6):559-568. DOI: 10.1007/s00737-014-0436-5

[35] Berit D, Pal R, Pal O, Lars J, Anne E. Placenta weight in pre-eclampsia. Acta Obstetricia et Gynecologica Scandinavica. 2008;**87**(6):608-611

[36] Lacobellia S, Bonsantea F, Robillard P. Pre-eclampsia and preterm birth in Reunion island: A 13 years cohort based study. Comparison with international data. Journal of Maternal-Fetal and Neonatal Medicine. 2016;**29**(18):3035-3040. DOI: 10.3109/14767058.2015.1114081

[37] Royal College of Obstetricians and Gynaecologists. The Management of Severe Pre-eclampsia/Eclampsia; National Institute for Health and Clinical Excellence (2008) Antenatal Care. NICE Clinical Guideline 62. London: National Institute for Health and Clinical Excellence; 2006

[38] Brian MM. Preterm premature rupture of the membranes: Diagnosis and management. Clinics in Perinatology. 2004;**31**(4):765-782

[39] Ahmed A, Rahman M, Zhang X, Acevedo CH, Nijjar S, Rushton I, et al. Induction of placental heme oxygenase-1 is protective against TNFalpha-induced cytotoxicity promotes vessel relaxation. Molecular Medicine. 2000;**6**:391-409

[40] George EM, Stout JM, Stec DE, Granger JP. Heme oxygenase induction attenuates TNF-α-induced hypertension in pregnant rodents. Frontiers in Pharmacology. 2015;**6**:165. DOI: 10.3389/fphar.2015.00165

[41] Kalantaridou SN, Zoumakis E, Makrigiannakis A, Lavasidis LG, Vrekoussis T, Chrousos GP. Corticotropin-releasing hormone, stress and humanreproduction: An update. Journal of Reproductive Immunology. 2010;**85**:33-39

[42] Wadhwa PD, Garite T, Porto M, Sandman CA. Corticotropin-releasing hormone (CRH), preterm birth and fetal growth restriction: A prospective investigation. American Journal of Obstetrics and Gynecology. 2004;**191**(4):1063-1069

[43] Keller PA, Kirkwood K, Morgan J, Westcott S, McCluskey A. The prevention of preterm labour—Corticotropin releasing hormone type 1 receptors as a target for drug design and development. Mini-Reviews in Medicinal Chemistry. 2016;**3**(4):295-303

[44] Torricelli M, Petraglia F. Placental hormones and identification of pregnancy at risk. Gynecological Endocrinology. 2010;**26**:705-707

[45] Voltolini C, Petraglia F. Neuroendocrinology of pregnancy and parturition. Clinical Neuroendocrinology. 2014;**124**:17-36. DOI: 10.1016/B978-0-444-59602-4.00002-2.

[46] Berghella V, Figueroa D, Szychowski JM, et al. 17-alpha-hydroxyprogesterone caproate for the prevention of preterm birth in women with prior preterm birth and a short cervical length. American Journal of Obstetrics and Gynecology. 2010;**202**(4):351, e1-6

[47] Committee on Practice Bulletins-The American College of Obstetricians and Gynecologists. Practice bulletin no. 130: Prediction and prevention of preterm birth. Obstetrics and Gynecology. 2012;**120**(4):964-973

[48] Dodd JM, Jones L, Flenady V, Cincotta R, Crowther CA. Prenatal administration of progesterone for preventing preterm birth in women considered to be at risk of preterm birth. Cochrane Database of Systematic Reviews. 2013;**7**:CD004947. DOI: 10.1002/14651858

[49] Tita ATN, Andrews WW. Diagnosis and management of clinical chorioamnionitis. Clinics in Perinatology. 2010;**37**(2):339-354

[50] Kadhim HJ, Duchateau J, Sebire G. Cytokines and brain injury: Invited review. Journal of Intensive Care Medicine. 2008;**23**:236-249

[51] Dammann O, Leviton A. Inflammatory brain damage in preterm newborns—Dry numbers, wet lab, and causal inferences. Early Human Development. 2004;**79**:1-15

[52] Malaeb S, Dammann O. Fetal inflammatory response and brain injury in the preterm newborn. Journal of Child Neurology. 2009;**24**(9):1119-1126

[53] Sciaky-Tamir Y, Hershkovitz R, Mazor M, Shelef I, Erez O. The use of imaging technology in the assessment of the fetal inflammatory response syndrome—Imaging of the fetal thymus. Prenatal Diagnosis. 2015;**35**(5):413-419

[54] Viscardi RM. Perinatal inflammation and lung injury. Seminars in Fetal & Neonatal Medicine. 2012;**17**(1):30-35

[55] Hoang M, Potter JA, Gysler SM, Han CS, Guller S, Norwitz ER, et al. Human fetal membranes generate distinct cytokine profiles in response to bacterial Toll-like receptor and nod-like receptor agonists. Biology of Reproduction. 2014;**90**(2):39

[56] Paananen R, Husa AK, Vuolteenaho R, Herva R, Kaukola T, Hallman M. Blood cytokines during the perinatal period in very preterm infants: Relationship of inflammatory response and bronchopulmonary dysplasia. The Journal of Pediatrics. 2009;**154**(39-43):e33

[57] Adams W, Rubens CE, Gravett MG. Use of nonhuman primate models to investigate mechanisms of infection-associated preterm birth. BJOG. 2011;**118**:136-144

[58] DiGiulio DB, Gervasi MT, Romero R, Vaisbuch E, Mazaki-Tovi S, Kusanovic JP, et al. Microbial invasion of the amniotic cavity in pregnancies with small-for-gestational-age fetuses. Journal of Perinatal Medicine. 2010a;**38**:495-502

[59] Bowes WA. The role of antibiotics in the prevention of preterm birth. F1000 Medicine Reports. 2009;**1**:22

[60] Bookstaver PB, Bland CM, Griffin B, Stover KR, Eiland LS, McLaughlin M. A review of antibiotic use in pregnancy. Pharmacotherapy: The Journal of Human Pharmacology and Drug Therapy. 2015;**35**(11):1052-1062

[61] Smaill F, Vazquez JC. Antibiotics for Asymptomatic Bacteriuria in

Pregnancy (Review). Cochrane Database Syst Rev. 7 Aug 2015;(8):CD000490. DOI: 10.1002/14651858.CD000490.pub3. Update in: Cochrane Database Syst Rev. 25 Nov 2019;**2019**(11). PMID: 26252501.

[62] Thinkhamrop J, Hofmeyr GJ, Adetoro O, Lumbiganon P. Prophylactic antibiotic administration in pregnancy to prevent infectious morbidity and mortality. Cochrane database of systematic reviews (online). 2002;**4**(4):cd002250

[63] Locksmith G, Duff P. Infection, antibiotics, and preterm delivery. Seminars in Perinatology. 2001;**25**(5):295-309

[64] Morency A, Bujold E. The effect of second-trimester antibiotic therapy on the rate of preterm birth. JOGC. 2007;**29**(1):35-44

[65] Simcox R, Sin WT, Seed PT, Briley A, Shennan AH. Prophylactic antibiotics for the prevention of preterm birth in women at risk: A meta-analysis. The Australian & New Zealand Journal of Obstetrics & Gynaecology. 2007;**47**:368-377

[66] Farag AH, Mohammed MM, Ellaithy MI, Salama HA. Blind vaginal fetal fibronectin swab for prediction of preterm birth. Journal of Obstetrics and Gynaecology Research. 2015;**41**(7):1009-1017

[67] Kiefer DG, Vintzileos AM. The utility of Fetal fibronectin in the prediction and prevention of spontaneous preterm birth. Reviews in Obstetrics and Gynecology. 2008;**1**(3):106-112

[68] Brian MM, Yolanda AR, Gary RT, Menachem MR, Robert LG, Anita FD, et al. The NICHD-MFMU antibiotic treatment of preterm PROM study: Impact of initial amniotic fluid volume on pregnancy outcome. American Journal of Obstetrics and Gynecology. 2006;**194**(2):438-445

[69] Joy S. Nichd Mfmu Network. Latency and infectious complications following preterm premature rupture of the membranes: Impact of body mass index. American Journal of Obstetrics and Gynecology. 2009;**201**(6):600.e1-5. DOI: 10.1016/j.ajog.2009.06.030

[70] Mercer BM, Crouse DT, Goldenberg RL, Miodovnik M, Mapp DC, Meis PJ, et al. The antibiotic treatment of PPROM study: Systemic maternal and fetal markers and perinatal outcomes. American Journal of Obstetrics and Gynecology. 2012;**206**(2):145.e1-145.e9

[71] Harirah H, Donita SE, Hsu CD. Amniotic fluid matrix metallo proteinase-9 and interleukin-6 in predicting intra-amniotic infection. Obstetrics and Gynecology. 2002;**99**:80-85

[72] Lee SE, Romero R, Jung H, Park CW, Park JS, Yoon BH. The intensity of the fetal inflammatory response in intraamniotic inflammation with and without microbial invasion of the amniotic cavity. American Journal of Obstetrics and Gynecology. 2007;**197**(294):e1-294.e6

[73] Taylor BD, Holzman CB, Fichorova RN, Tian Y, Jones NM, Wenjiang F, et al. Inflammation biomarkers in vaginal fluid and preterm delivery. Human Reproduction. 2013;**28**(4):942-952

[74] O'Brien CM, Arbuckle S, Thomas S, Rode J, Turner R, Jeffery HE. Placental inflammation is associated with rural and remote residence in the Northern Territory, Australia: A cross-sectional study. BMC Pregnancy and Childbirth. 2015;**15**:32

[75] Lee SE, Romero R, Park CW, Jun JK, Yoon BH. The frequency and significance

of intraamniotic inflammation in patients with cervical insufficiency. American Journal of Obstetrics and Gynecology. 2008;**198**:633.e1-633.e8

[76] Queenan JT, Spong CY, Lockwood CJ. Protocols for High-Risk Pregnancies: An Evidence-Based Approach. Wiley-Blackwell. Available from: https://doi.org/10.1002/9781444323870

[77] Suhag A, Berghella V. Cervical cerclage. Clinical Obstetrics and Gynecology. 2014;**57**(3):557-567

[78] Kristen L, Camilo A, Clinton J, Nelson M, Brian M, Cameron MJ, et al. Differential receptor for advanced glycation end products expression in preeclamptic, intrauterine growth restricted, and gestational diabetic placentas. American Journal of Reproductive Immunology. 2016;**75**(2):172-180

[79] Rzepka R, Dołegowska B, Rajewska A, Kwiatkowski S, Sałata D, Budkowska M, et al. Soluble and endogenous secretory receptors for advanced glycation end products in threatened preterm labor and preterm premature rupture of fetal membranes. BioMed Research International. 2015;**2015**; Article ID 568042, p. 10

[80] Schaefer TM, Desouza K, Fahey JV, Beagley KW, Wira CR. Toll-like receptor (TLR) expression and TLR-mediated cytokine/chemokine production by human uterine epithelial cells. Immunology. 2004;**112**(3):428-436

[81] Buhimschi IA, Zhao G, Pettker CM. The receptor for advanced glycation end products (RAGE) system in women with intraamniotic infection and inflammation. American Journal of Obstetrics and Gynecology. 2007;**196**(181):e1-181.e12

[82] Dubicke A, Andersson P, Fransson E, Andersson E, Sioutas A, et al. High-mobility group box protein 1 and its signalling receptors in human preterm and term cervix. Journal of Reproductive Immunology. 2010;**84**(1):86-94

[83] Thaxton JE, Nevers TA, Sharma S. TLR-mediated preterm birth in response to pathogenic agents. Infectious Diseases in Obstetrics and Gynecology. 2010;**2010**, pii: 378472

[84] Noguchi T, Sado T, Naruse K, Shigetomi H, Onogi A, Haruta S, et al. Evidence for activation of Toll-like receptor and receptor for advanced glycation end products in preterm birth. Mediators of Inflammation. 2010:1-10. Article ID 490406

[85] Bastek JA, Brown AG, Foreman MN, McShea MA, Anglim LM, Adamczak JE, et al. The soluble receptor for advanced glycation end products can prospectively identify patients at greatest risk for preterm birth. The Journal of Maternal-Fetal & Neonatal Medicine. 2012;**25**:1762-1768

[86] Romero R, Chaiworapongsa T, Savasan ZA, Hussein Y, Dong Z, Kusanovic JP, et al. Clinical chorioamnionitis is characterized by changes in the expression of the alarmin HMGB1 and one of its receptors, sRAGE. The Journal of Maternal-Fetal & Neonatal Medicine. 2012;**25**:558-567

[87] Bezold KY, Karjalainen MK, Hallman M, Teramo K, Muglia LJ. The genomics of preterm birth: From animal models to human studies. Genome Medicine. 2013;**5**:34

[88] Krediet TG, Wiertsema SP, Vossers MJ, Hoeks SBEA, Fleer A, Ruven HJT, et al. Toll-like receptor 2 polymorphism is associated with preterm birth. Pediatric Research. 2007;**62**(4):474-476

[89] Espinoza J. Uteroplacental ischemia in early- and late-onset

pre-eclampsia: A role for the fetus? Ultrasound in Obstetrics & Gynecology. 2012;**40**(4):373-382

[90] Gilbert JS, Bauer AJ, Gingery A, Chasson S. Circulating and utero-placental adaptations to chronic placental ischemia in the rat. Placenta. 2011;**33**(2):100-105

[91] Granger JP, Alexander BT, Llinas MT, Bennett WA, Khalil RA. Pathophysiology of preeclampsia: Linking placental ischemia/hypoxia with microvascular dysfunction. Microcirculation. 2002;**9**(3):147-160

[92] Thompson RJ, Goldstein RF, Oehler JM, Gustafson KE, Catlett AT, Brazy JE. Developmental outcome of very low birth weight infants as a function of biological risk and psychosocial risk. Journal of Developmental and Behavioral Pediatrics. 1994;**15**(4):232-238

[93] Van Ierssе SH, Conraads VM, Van Craenenbroeck EM, Liu Y, Maas A, Parizel PM, et al. Endothelial dysfunction in acute brain injury and the development of cerebral ischemia. Journal of Neuroscience Research. 2015;**93**(6):866-872

[94] Livrinova V, Hadzi Lega M, Hristova Dimcheva A, Samardziski I, Isjanovska R. Factor V Leiden, prothrombin and MTHFR mutation in patients with Preeclamsia, intrauterine growth restriction and placental abruption. Open Access Macedonian Journal of Medical Sciences. DOI: 10.3889/oamjms.2015.099

[95] Chighizola CB, Andreoli L, de Jesus GR, Banzato A, Pons-Estel GJ, Erkan D. The association between antiphospholipid antibodies and pregnancy morbidity, stroke, myocardial infarction, and deep vein thrombosis: A critical review of the literature. Lupus. 2015;**24**:980-984

[96] Giancotti A, La Torre R, Spagnuolo A, D'Ambrosio V, Cerekja A, Piazze J. Efficacy of three different antithrombotic regimens on pregnancy outcome in pregnant women affected by recurrent pregnancy loss. The Journal of Maternal-Fetal & Neonatal Medicine. 2012;**25**(7):1191-1194

[97] Karakantza M, Androutsopoulos G, Mougiou A, Decavalas GO. Inheritance and perinatal consequences of inherited thrombophilia in Greece. International Journal of Gynecology & Obstetrics. 2008;**100**(2):124-129

[98] Dhobale M, Chavan P, Kulkarni A, Mehendale S, Pisal H, Joshi S. Reduced folate, increased vitamin B(12) and homocysteine concentrations in women delivering preterm. Annals of Nutrition and Metabolism. 2012;**61**:7-14

[99] Bergen NE, Jaddoe VWV, Timmermans S, et al. Homocysteine and folate concentrations in early pregnancy and the risk of adverse pregnancy outcomes: The generation R study. British Journal of Obstetrics and Gynaecology. 2012;**119**(6):739-751

[100] Blencowe H, Cousens S, Oestergaard M, Chou D, Moller AB, Narwal R, et al. National, regional and worldwide estimates of preterm birth. The Lancet. 2012;**379**(9832):2162-2172

[101] Charles DHM, Ness AR, Campbell D, Smith GD, Whitley E, Hall MH. Folic acid supplements in pregnancy and birth outcome: Re-analysis of a large randomised controlled trial and update of Cochrane review. Paediatric and Perinatal Epidemiology. 2005;**19**(2):112-124

[102] Lee J, Romero R, Xu Y, Kim JS, Topping V, Yoo W, et al. A signature

of maternal anti-fetal rejection in spontaneous preterm birth: Chronic chorioamnionitis, anti-human leukocyte antigen antibodies, and C4d. PLoS One. 2011;**6**(2):e16806

[103] Young RC. Synchronization of regional contractions of human labor; direct effects of region size and tissue excitability. Journal of Biomechanics. 2015;**48**(9):1614-1619

[104] Lucovnik M, Kuon RJ, Chambliss LR, Maner WL, Shi S, Leili Shi L, et al. Progestin treatment for the prevention of preterm birth. Acta Obstetricia et Gynecologica Scandinavica. 2011;**90**(10):1057-1069

[105] Romero R, Yeo L, Chaemsaithong P, Chaiworapongsa T, Hassan SS. Progesterone to prevent spontaneous preterm birth. Seminars in Fetal & Neonatal Medicine. 2014;**19**(1):15-26

[106] Zhang H, Zhang L. Role of protein kinase C isozymes in the regulation of alpha$_1$-adrenergic receptor-mediated contractions in ovine uterine arteries. Biology of Reproduction. 2008;**78**(1):35-42

[107] Xiao D, Longo LD, Zhang L. Alpha1-adrenoceptor-mediated phosphorylation of MYPT-1 and CPI-17 in the uterine artery: Role of ERK/PKC. American Journal of Physiology. Heart and Circulatory Physiology. 2005;**288**(6):H2828-H2835

[108] An BS, Ahn HJ, Kang HS, Jung EM, Yang H, Hong EJ, et al. Effects of estrogen and estrogenic compounds, 4-tert-octylphenol, and bisphenol A on the uterine contraction and contraction-associated proteins in rats. Molecular and Cellular Endocrinology. 2013;**375**(1-2):27-34

[109] Elmes M, Szyszka A, Pauliat C, Clifford B, Daniel Z, Cheng Z, et al. Maternal age effects on myometrial expression of contractile proteins, uterine gene expression, and contractile activity during labor in the rat. Physiological Reports. 2015;**3**(4):e12305

[110] Cook JL, Zaragoza DB, Sung DH, Olson DM. Expression of myometrial activation and stimulation genes in a mouse model of preterm labor: Myometrial activation, stimulation, and preterm labor. Endocrinology. 2000;**141**(5):1718-1728

[111] Chinnathambi V, Blesson CS, Vincent KL, Saade GR, Hankins GD, Yallampalli C, et al. Elevated testosterone levels during rat pregnancy cause hypersensitivity to angiotensin II and attenuation of endothelium-dependent vasodilation in uterine arteries. Hypertension. 2014;**64**:405-414

[112] Gokina NI, Kuzina OY, Vance AM. Augmented EDHF signaling in rat uteroplacental vasculature during late pregnancy. American Journal of Physiology. Heart and Circulatory Physiology. 2010;**299**:H1642-H1652

[113] Lee J, Romero R, Xu Y, Kim JS, Park JY, Kusanovic JP, et al. Maternal HLA panel-reactive antibodies in early gestation positively correlate with chronic chorioamnionitis: Evidence in support of the chronic nature of maternal anti-fetal rejection. American Journal of Reproductive Immunology. 2011;**66**(6):510-526

[114] Tirado-González I, Nancy Freitag N, Gabriela Barrientos G, Blois SM. Galectin-I influences trophoblast immune evasion and emerges as a predictive factor for the outcome of pregnancy. Molecular Human Reproduction. 2013;**19**(1):43-53

[115] Khashan AS, Kenny LS, Laursen TM, Mahmood U,

Mortensen PB, Henriksen TB, et al. Pregnancy and the risk of autoimmune disease. PLoS One. 2011;**6**(5):e19658

[116] Bytautiene E, Romero R, Vedernikov YP. Induction of premature labor and delivery by alergic reaction and prevention by histamin H1 receptor antagonist. American Journal of Obstetrics and Gynecology. 2004;**191**:1356-1361

[117] Williams Z. Inducing tolerance to pregnancy. New England Journal of Medicine. 2012;**367**:1159-1161

[118] Kar S, Krishnan A, Preetha K, Mohankar A. A review of antihistamines used during pregnancy. Journal of Pharmacology and Pharmacotherapeutics. 2012;**3**(2):105-108

[119] Adams Waldorf KM, Singh N, Mohan AR. Uterine overdistention induces preterm labor mediated by inflammation: Observations in pregnant women and nonhuman primates. American Journal of Obstetrics and Gynecology. 2015;**213**(830):e1-e19

[120] Lee YH, Shynlova O, Lye SJ. Stretchinduced human myometrial cytokines enhance immune cell recruitment via endothelial activation. Cellular & Molecular Immunology. 2015;**12**:231-242

[121] Davidson JO, Drury PP, Green CR, Nicholson LF, Bennet L, Gunn AJ. Connexin hemichannel blockade is neuroprotective after asphyxia in preterm fetal sheep. PLoS One. 2014;**9**(5):e96558

[122] Kirton A. Modeling developmental plasticity after perinatal stroke: Defining central therapeutic targets in cerebral palsy. Pediatric Neurology. 2013;**48**(2):81-94

[123] Sclowitz IK, Santos IS, Domingues MR, Matijasevich A, Barros AJ. Prognostic factors for low birthweight repetition in successive pregnancies: A cohort study. BMC Pregnancy and Childbirth. 2013;**13**:20. DOI: 10.1186/1471-2393-13-20

[124] Villar J, Giuliani F, Bhutta ZA, Bertino E, Ohuma EO, Ismail LC, et al. Postnatal growth standards for preterm infants: The preterm postnatal follow-up study of the INTERGROWTH-21(st) project. The Lancet Global Health. 2015;**3**(11):e681-e691

[125] Yee LM, Truong YN, Caughey AB, Cheng YW. The association between interdelivery interval and adverse perinatal outcomes in a diverse US population. Journal of Perinatology. 2016;**36**(8):593-597. DOI: 10.1038/jp.2016.54

[126] Lefebvre F, Gagnon MM, Luu TM, Lupien G, Dorval V. In extremely preterm infants, do the movement assessment of infants and the Alberta infant motor scale predict 18-month outcomes using the Bayley-III? Early Human Development. 2016;**94**:13-17. DOI: 10.1016/j.earlhumdev.2016.01.012

[127] Ramel SE, Demerath EW, Gray HL, Younge N, Boys C, Georgieff MK. The relationship of poor linear growth velocity with neonatal illness and two-year neurodevelopment in preterm infants. Neonatology. 2012;**102**(1):19-24

[128] Rimol LM, Bjuland KJ, Løhaugen GC, Martinussen M, Evensen KA, Indredavik MS, et al. Cortical trajectories during adolescence in preterm born teenagers with very low birthweight. Cortex. 2016;**75**:120-131. DOI: 10.1016/j.cortex.2015.12.001

[129] Doyle LW, Cheong JL, Burnett A, Roberts G, Lee KJ, Anderson PJ. Victorian infant collaborative study group.

Biological and social influences on outcomes of extreme-preterm/low-birth weight adolescents. Pediatrics. 2015;**136**(6):e1513-e1520

[130] Spittle A, Orton J, Anderson PJ, Boyd R, Doyle LW. Early developmental intervention programmes provided post hospital discharge to prevent motor and cognitive impairment in preterm infants. Cochrane Database of Systematic Reviews. 2015;**11**:CD005495. DOI: 10.1002/14651858

[131] Coq JO, Delcour M, Massicotte VS, Baud O, Barbe MF. Prenatal ischemia deteriorates white matter, brain organization, and function: Implications for prematurity and cerebral palsy. Developmental Medicine & Child Neurology. 2016;**58**(4):7-11

[132] Eneriz-Wiemer M, Saynina O, Sundaram V, Lee HC, Bhattacharya J, Sanders LM. Parent language: A predictor for neurodevelopmental follow-up care among infants with very low birth weight. Academic Pediatrics. 2016;**16**(7):645-52. DOI: 10.1016/j.acap.2016.04.004.

[133] Huseynova SA, Panakhova NF, Hajiyeva AS, Mukhtarova SN, Agayeva GT. Endothelial dysfunction and developmental outcomes of very low birth weight newborns with hypoxic encephalopathy. JPMA. 2017;**67**(12):1857-1863

[134] Ramoğlu M, Kavuncuoğlu S, Aldemir E, Yarar C, Eras Z. Neurodevelopment of preterms born after IVF and spontaneous multiple pregnancies. Pediatrics International. 2016;**58**(12)1284-1290. DOI: 10.1111/ped.13012

[135] Szczapa T, Karpiński Ł, Moczko J, Weindling M, Kornacka A, Wróblewska K, et al. Comparison of cerebral tissue oxygenation values in full term and preterm newborns by the simultaneous use of two near-infrared spectroscopy devices: An absolute and a relative trending oximeter. Journal of Biomedical Optics. 2013;**18**(8):87006. DOI: 10.1117/1.JBO.18.8.087006

[136] Haller S, Deindl P, Cassini A, Suetens C, Zingg W, Abu Sin M, et al. Neurological sequelae of healthcare-associated sepsis in very-low-birthweight infants: Umbrella review and evidence-based outcome tree. Euro Surveillance. 2016;**21**(8). DOI: 10.2807/1560-7917.ES.2016.21.8.30143

[137] Lee JY, Ahn TG, Jun JK. Short-term and long-term postnatal outcomes of expectant management after previable preterm premature rupture of membranes with and without persistent oligohydramnios. Obstetrics and Gynecology. 2015;**126**(5):947-953

[138] Milner KM, Neal EF, Roberts G, Steer AC, Duke T. Long-term neurodevelopmental outcome in high-risk newborns in resource-limited settings: A systematic review of the literature. Paediatrics and International Child Health. 2015;**35**(3):227-242

[139] Miyazaki K, Furuhashi M, Ishikawa K, Tamakoshi K, Hayashi K, Kai A, et al. Impact of chorioamnionitis on short- and long-term outcomes in very low birth weight preterm infants: The Neonatal Research Network Japan. The Journal of Maternal-Fetal & Neonatal Medicine. 2016;**29**(2):331-337

[140] Radic JA, Vincer M, McNeely PD. Outcomes of intraventricular hemorrhage and posthemorrhagic hydrocephalus in a population-based cohort of very preterm infants born to residents of Nova Scotia from 1993 to 2010. Journal of Neurosurgery. Pediatrics. 2015;**15**(6):580-588

[141] Wu T, Fan XP, Wang WY, Yuan TM. Enterovirus infections are associated

with white matter damage in neonates. Journal of Paediatrics and Child Health. 2014;**50**(10):817-822

[142] Li D, Hodge J, Wei XC, Kirton A. Reduced ipsilesional cortical volumes in fetal periventricular venous infarction. Stroke. 2012;**43**(5):1404-1407

[143] Pappas A, Kendrick DE, Shankaran S, Stoll BJ, Bell EF, Laptook AR, et al. Eunice Kennedy Shriver National Institute of Child Health and Human Development Neonatal Research Network. Chorioamnionitis and early childhood outcomes among extremely low-gestational-age neonates. JAMA Pediatrics. 2014;**168**(2):137-147

[144] Stoll BJ, Hansen NI, Bell EF, Walsh MC, Carlo WA, Shankaran S, et al. Trends in care practices, morbidity, and mortality of extremely preterm neonates, 1993-2012. Journal of the American Medical Association. 2015;**314**(10):1039-1051

[145] Jary S, Kmita G, Wroblewska J, Whitelaw A. Quantitative cranial ultrasound prediction of severity of disability in premature infants with post-haemorrhagic ventricular dilatation. Archives of Disease in Childhood. 2012;**97**:955-959

[146] Ramenghi LA, Fumagalli M, Righini A, Bassi L, Groppo M, Parazzini C, et al. Magnetic resonance imaging assessment of brain maturation in preterm neonates with punctate white matter lesions. Neuroradiology. 2007;**49**:161-167

[147] Smyser CD, Kidokoro H, Inder TE. Magnetic resonance imaging of the brain at term equivalent age in extremely premature neonates: To scan or not to scan? Journal of Paediatrics and Child Health. 2012;**48**:794-800

[148] Lee W, Al-Dossary H, Raybaud C, Young JM, Morgan BR, Whyte HE, et al. Longitudinal cerebellar growth following very preterm birth. Journal of Magnetic Resonance Imaging. 2016;**43**(6):1462-1473. DOI: 10.1002/jmri.25098

[149] Navarra R, Sestieri C, Conte E, Salomone R, Mattei PA, Romani GL, et al. Perinatal MRI diffusivity is related to early assessment of motor performance in preterm neonates. The Neuroradiology Journal. 2016;**29**(2):137-145

[150] Arichi T, Counsell SJ, Allievi AG, Chew AT, Martinez-Biarge M, Mondi V, et al. The effects of hemorrhagic parenchymal infarction on the establishment of sensori-motor structural and functional connectivity in early infancy. Neuroradiology. 2014;**56**(11):985-994

[151] Kidokoro H, Anderson PJ, Doyle LW, Woodward LJ, Neil JJ, Inder TE. Brain injury and altered brain growth in preterm infants: Predictors and prognosis. Pediatrics. 2014;**134**(2):e444-e453

[152] Merchant N, Azzopardi D. Early predictors of outcome in infants treated with hypothermia for hypoxic-ischaemic encephalopathy. Developmental Medicine and Child Neurology. 2015;**57**(Suppl. 3):8-16

[153] Massaro AN, Evangelou I, Fatemi A, Vezina G, Mccarter R, Glass P, et al. White matter tract integrity and developmental outcome in newborn infants with hypoxic-ischemic encephalopathy treated with hypothermia. Developmental Medicine and Child Neurology. 2015;**57**(5):441-448

[154] Thompson DK, Chen J, Beare R, Adamson CL, Ellis R, Ahmadzai ZM,

et al. Structural connectivity relates to perinatal factors and functional impairment at 7years in children born very preterm. NeuroImage. 2016;**134**:328-337

[155] Setänen S, Haataja L, Parkkola R, Lehtonen L, Lind A. Predictive value of neonatal brain MRI on the neurodevelopmental outcome of preterm infants by 5 years of age. Acta Paediatrica. 2013;**102**:492-497

[156] Lind A, Haataja L, Rautava L, Valiaho A, Lehtonen L, Lapinleimu H, et al. Relations between brain volumes, neuropsychological assessment and parental questionnaire in prematurely born children. European Child & Adolescent Psychiatry. 2010;**19**:407-417

[157] Sølsnes AE, Sripada K, Yendiki A, Bjuland K, Østgård HF, Aanes S, et al. Limited microstructural and connectivity deficits despite subcortical volume reductions in school-aged children born preterm with very low birth weight. NeuroImage. 2016;**130**:24-34

[158] Rahmati H, Martens H, Aamo OM, Stavdahl Ø, Støen R, Adde L. Frequency-based features for early cerebral palsy prediction. Conference Proceedings: Annual International Conference of the IEEE Engineering in Medicine and Biology Society. 2015;**2015**:5187-5190. DOI: 10.1109/EMBC.2015.7319560

[159] Strand KM, Dahlseng MO, Lydersen S, Rø TB, Finbråten AK, Jahnsen RB, et al. Growth during infancy and early childhood in children with cerebral palsy: A population-based study. Developmental Medicine and Child Neurology. 2016;**58**(9):924-30. DOI: 10.1111/dmcn.13098

[160] Verma R, Shibly S, Fang H, Pollack S. Do early postnatal body weight changes contribute to neonatal morbidities in the extremely low birth weight infants. Journal of Neonatal-Perinatal Medicine. 2015;**8**(2):113-118

[161] Bhatt AJ, Feng Y, Wang J, Famuyide M, Hersey K. Dexamethasone induces apoptosis of progenitor cells in the subventricular zone and dentate gyrus of developing rat brain. Journal of Neuroscience Research. 2013;**91**(9):1191-1202

[162] Linsell L, Malouf R, Morris J, Kurinczuk JJ, Marlow N. Prognostic factors for cerebral palsy and motor impairment in children born very preterm or very low birthweight: A systematic review. Developmental Medicine and Child Neurology. 2015:**169**(12):1162-1172. DOI: 10.1111/dmcn.12972

[163] Zia MT, Vinukonda G, Vose LR, Bhimavarapu BB, Iacobas S, Pandey NK, et al. Postnatal glucocorticoid-induced hypomyelination, gliosis, and neurologic deficits are dose-dependent, preparation-specific, and reversible. Experimental Neurology. 2015;**263**:200-213

[164] Schieve LA, Tian LH, Rankin K, Kogan MD, Yeargin-Allsopp M, Visser S, et al. Population impact of preterm birth and low birth weight on developmental disabilities in US children. Annals of Epidemiology. 2016;**26**(4):267-274

[165] Slaughter LA, Bonfante-Mejia E, Hintz SR, Dvorchik I, Parikh NA. Early conventional MRI for prediction of neurodevelopmental impairment in extremely-low-birth-weight infants. Neonatology. 2016;**110**(1):47-54

[166] Bolduc ME, Du Plessis AJ, Sullivan N, Khwaja OS, Zhang X, Barnes K, et al. Spectrum of neurodevelopmental disabilities in children with cerebellar malformations. Developmental Medicine and Child Neurology. 2011;**53**(5):409-416

[167] Greiner MV, Lawrence AP, Horn P, Newmeyer AJ, Makoroff KL. Early clinical indicators of developmental outcome in abusive head trauma. Child's Nervous System. 2012;**28**(6):889-896

[168] Marete I, Tenge C, Pasha O, Goudar S, Chomba E, Patel A, et al. Perinatal outcomes of multiple-gestation pregnancies in Kenya, Zambia, Pakistan, India, Guatemala, and Argentina: A global network study. American Journal of Perinatology. 2014;**31**(2):125-132

[169] Nath S, Roy R, Mukherjee S. Perinatal complications associated with autism—A case control study in a neurodevelopment and early intervention clinic. Journal of the Indian Medical Association. 2012;**110**(8):526-529

[170] François C, Ripollés P, Bosch L, Garcia-Alix A, Muchart J, Sierpowska J, et al. Language learning and brain reorganization in a 3.5-year-old child with left perinatal stroke revealed using structural and functional connectivity. Cortex. 2016;**77**:95-118

[171] Young JM, Powell TL, Morgan BR, Card D, Lee W, Smith ML, et al. Deep grey matter growth predicts neurodevelopmental outcomes in very preterm children. NeuroImage. 2015;**111**:360-368. DOI: 10.1016/j.neuroimage.2015.02.030. Epub 2015 Feb 21

[172] Roberts G, Cheong J, Opie G, et al. Growth of extremely preterm survivors from birth to 18 years of age compared with term controls. Pediatrics. 2013;**131**(2):e439-e445. DOI: 10.1542/peds.2012-1135.

[173] Bocca-Tjeertes IFA, Kerstjens JM, Reijneveld SA, de Winter AF, Bos AF. Growth and predictors of growth restraint in moderately preterm children aged 0 to 4 years. Pediatrics. 2011;**128**(5):e1187-e1194. DOI: 10.1542/peds.2010-3781

[174] Bayer JK, Hiscock H, Ukoumunne OC, Price A, Wake M. Early childhood aetiology of mental health problems: A longitudinal population-based study. Journal of Child Psychology and Psychiatry. 2008;**49**(11):1166-1174

[175] Huhtala M, Korja R, Lehtonen L, Haataja L, Lapinleimu H, Rautava P. Parental psychological well-being and behavioral outcome of very low birth weight infants at 3 years. Pediatrics. 2012;**129**(4):937-945

[176] Embleton ND, Skeath T. Catch-up growth and metabolic and cognitive outcomes in adolescents born preterm. Nestle Nutrition Institute Workshop Series. 2015;**81**:61-71

[177] Teller IC, Embleton ND, Griffin IJ, van Elburg RM. Post-discharge formula feeding in preterm infants: A systematic review mapping evidence about the role of macronutrient enrichment. Clinical Nutrition. 2015. pii: S0261-5614(15)00227-7. DOI: 10.1016/j.clnu.2015.08.006

[178] Schmidt B, Roberts RS, Davis PG, et al. Prediction of late death or disability at age 5 years using a count of 3 neonatal morbidities in very low birth weight infants. The Journal of Pediatrics. 2015;**167**:982

[179] Casolini P, Zuena AR, et al. Sub-neurotoxic neonatal anoxia induces subtle behavioural changes and specific abnormalities in brain group-I metabotropic glutamate receptors in rats. Journal of Neurochemistry. 2005;**95**:137-145

[180] Padilla VT et al. Impact of severe intrauterine restriction on

brain development. Acta Paediatrica. 2009;**98**(suppl. 460):204

[181] Bjuland KJ, Rimol LM, Løhaugen GC, Skranes J. Brain volumes and cognitive function in very-low-birth-weight (VLBW) young adults. European Journal of Paediatric Neurology. 2014;**18**(5):578-590

[182] Botellero VL, Skranes J, Bjuland KJ, Løhaugen GC, Håberg AK, Lydersen S, et al. Mental health and cerebellar volume during adolescence in very-low-birth-weight infants: A longitudinal study. Child and Adolescent Psychiatry and Mental Health. 2016;**10**:6. DOI: 10.1186/s13034-016-0093-8

[183] Lees C, Marlow N, Arabin B, Bilardo CM, Brezinka C, Derks JB, et al. Perinatal morbidity and mortality in early-onset fetal growth restriction: Cohort outcomes of the trial of randomized umbilical and fetal flow in Europe (TRUFFLE). Ultrasound in Obstetrics & Gynecology. 2013;**42**:400-408

[184] Pham H, Duy AP, Pansiot J, Bollen B, Gallego J, Charriaut-Marlangue C, et al. Impact of inhaled nitric oxide on white matter damage in growth-restricted neonatal rats. Pediatric Research. 2015;77(4):563-569

[185] Hauglann L, Handegaard BH, Ulvund SE, Nordhov M, Rønning JA, Kaaresen PI. Cognitive outcome of early intervention in preterms at 7 and 9 years of age: A randomised controlled trial. Archives of Disease in Childhood. Fetal and Neonatal Edition. 2015;**100**(1):F11-F16

[186] Van Wassenaer-Leemhuis AG, Jeukens-Visser M, van Hus JW, Meijssen D, Wolf MJ, Kok JH, et al. Rethinking preventive post-discharge intervention programmes for very preterm infants and their parents. Developmental Medicine and Child Neurology. 2016;**58**(Suppl 4):67-73

[187] Swamy MK, Kamal P, Shailaja N. Maternal and perinatal outcome during expectant management. The Journal of Obstetrics and Gynecology of India. 2012;**62**(4):413-418